Substance Abuse:
A Guide for
Health Professionals

American Academy of Pediatrics
(AAP)

Center for Advanced Health
Studies (CAHS)

This book is made possible
by grants from
IBM Corporation
and
The Pew Charitable Trusts

Library of Congress Catalog Number 88-72274
ISBN 0-910761-20-5

Quantity prices available on request. Address all inquiries to:

American Academy of Pediatrics
141 Northwest Point Boulevard
P.O. Box 927
Elk Grove Village, IL 60009-0927

Contributors and Consultants

The chapters of this guide have no specific authors; contributors were responsible for preparing initial drafts of chapters. Subsequently, these initial drafts were submitted to consultants as well as to members of the editorial and advisory boards. Opinions of all reviewers were considered by the editors in the preparation of the final manuscript. The work of the following contributors and consultants was essential to the evolution of this guide:

Michael I. Cohen, MD
Professor and Chairman
Department of Pediatrics
Montefiore Medical Center
Albert Einstein College of Medicine
Bronx, New York

Shirley D. Coletti
Executive Director
Operation PAR, Inc. (Parental Awareness and
    Responsibility)
Immediate Past Chairman of the National Federation
    of Parents for Drug Free Youth
Pinellas Park, Florida

Susan M. Coupey, MD
Associate Director, Division of Adolescent Medicine
Montefiore Medical Center
Associate Professor of Pediatrics
Albert Einstein College of Medicine
Bronx, New York

George D. Comerci, MD, FAAP
Chief, Adolescent and Young Adult Medicine
University of Arizona College of Medicine
Professor, Pediatrics and Family Medicine
Tucson, Arizona

Dorynne Czechowicz, MD
Associate Director for Medical and Professional Affairs
National Institute on Drug Abuse
Office of Science
Rockville, Maryland

Nancy Neveloff Dubler, LL.B.
Director, Division of Legal and Ethical Issues
  in Health Care
Montefiore Medical Center
Associate Professor of Epidemiology and Social Medicine
Albert Einstein College of Medicine
Bronx, New York

Marianne E. Felice, MD
Chief, Division of Adolescent Medicine
University of California San Diego Medical Center
Associate Professor of Pediatrics
University of California San Diego School of Medicine
San Diego, California

Vincent A. Fulginiti, MD
Acting Dean and Senior Vice-Dean for Academic Affairs
Professor of Pediatrics
University of Arizona College of Medicine
Tucson, Arizona
Chairman, AAP Task Force on Substance Abuse (1985)

Michael D. Klitzner, PhD
Project Director
Health Professionals as Preventors
Pacific Institute for Research and Evaluation
Vienna, Virginia

John E. Meeks, MD
Medical Director
Psychiatric Institute of Montgomery County
Rockville, Maryland

Walter D. Rosenfeld, MD
Director, Adolescent Ambulatory Service
Montefiore Medical Center
Assistant Professor of Pediatrics
Albert Einstein College of Medicine
Bronx, New York

S. Kenneth Schonberg, MD
Director, Division of Adolescent Medicine
Montefiore Medical Center
Professor of Pediatrics
Albert Einstein College of Medicine
Bronx, New York

Richard H. Schwartz, MD
Clinical Professor of Child Health and Development
George Washington University School of Medicine
Washington, DC
Clinical Assistant Professor of Family Medicine
Medical College of Virginia
Richmond, Virginia

Arnold M. Washton, PhD
Executive Director
The Washton Institute
Outpatient Addiction Treatment Centers
New York, New York

AAP Task Force on Substance Abuse

George D. Comerci, MD, Chairman (1985-1987)
Vincent A. Fulginiti, MD, Chairman (1985)
Albert W. Pruitt, MD
S. Kenneth Schonberg, MD
Richard H. Schwartz, MD
William C. Van Ost, MD

Consultant
Joe M. Sanders, Jr., MD

AAP Provisional Committee on Substance Abuse

Albert W. Pruitt, MD, Chairman (1987-present)
Edward A. Jacobs, MD
Manuel Schydlower, MD, Col MC, US Army
Benjamin O. Stands, MD
Jonathan M. Sutton, MD

Center for Advanced Health Studies Advisory Panel

Margaret Blasinsky
Center for Advanced Health Studies

Allan Y. Cohen, PhD
Pacific Institute for Research and Evaluation

Shirley D. Coletti
Operation PAR (Parental Awareness and Responsibility)

George D. Comerci, MD
American Academy of Pediatrics

Dorynne Czechowicz, MD
National Institute on Drug Abuse

Robert L. Dupont, MD
Center for Behavioral Medicine

John J. Graham, MD
American College of Obstetricians and Gynecologists

Michael D. Klitzner, PhD
Pacific Institute for Research and Evaluation

Daniel J. Ostergaard, MD
American Academy of Family Physicians

Robert Prentice, MD
American Academy of Pediatrics

S. Kenneth Schonberg, MD
American Academy of Pediatrics

Tomas Silber, MD
Children's Hospital National Medical Center

Bonnie Wilford
American Medical Association

The Editorial Board expresses appreciation to Carole
Corbett, Maureen DeRosa, and Jean D. Lockhart,
M.D. of the American Academy of Pedicatrics; Liese
A. Scribner and Sally H. Thoureen of the Center for
Advanced Health Studies; and Linda R. Harteker,
Medical Editor.

Dedication

This guide is dedicated to the youth of our nation, who are, in the main, good people representing the very best we as parents, educators, and health professionals are able to produce. They are, nevertheless, inheritors of a culture in which the dangers of drug abuse are ever present and therefore need and deserve our best efforts to assist them in the journey toward a healthy, productive adulthood. And to ourselves, we owe the reassurance of knowing that when we are ready to pass responsibility to the next generation, that generation will be optimally prepared to receive it.

Table of Contents

PREFACE

THE PROBLEM

The use of psychoactive drugs by children and adolescents represents an urgent societal problem: this fact is no longer questioned. In recent years, substance abuse by young people has become the focus of national attention, and programs to prevent drug use, minimize the consequences of use, and treat abusers have been widely publicized. Despite this publicity, however, we have not yet mobilized the majority of health professionals toward effective intervention.

Many obstacles stand in the way of effective intervention. Among the more difficult of these are disagreements as to the nature of effective intervention. Is the task to prevent drug use, to postpone such use, or to minimize the consequences of "inevitable" or "normative" use? Or is it all of the above? Whose job is it? Should drug abuse be a primary concern for physicians and other health professionals? Is it not more appropriately an issue for parents, educators, clergy, the police, business and industry, and legislators?

Such questions often do little more than camouflage more important impediments to action. Behavioral intervention is frequently more difficult, more complex, and less likely to produce rapid and tangible results than time spent addressing physiologic dysfunction. Preventing drug use or its consequences is not only time-consuming; it also requires interviewing techniques, treatment approaches, counseling skills, and a knowledge base that may be missing from the practitioner's armamentarium. Providing the basis for such techniques, approaches, skills, and knowledge serves as the motivation for this guide.

THE DATA

More than 90% of adolescents in the United States will have used alcohol before graduating from high school, and two thirds of seniors report drinking in the past month. Fifty percent of seniors report having ever used marijuana, and one fourth of seniors report having used it in the last 30 days. Approximately 5% of seniors use either marijuana or alcohol daily (Table 1). Alcohol and marijuana use began before entrance to high school for approximately 30% and 10%, respectively, of seniors (Table 2).[1] These data are somewhat conservative, as those young people who had left school before their senior year would not have been included within these surveys and as drug use among this population of "drop-outs" is probably higher than that encountered among their in-school peers.

Table 1
Drug Use by High School Seniors—Class of 1986
(in percent)

	EVER USED	PAST MONTH	DAILY
Alcohol	91	66	5
Marijuana	51	23	4
Cocaine	17	5	0.2
Hallucinogens	12	4	0.3
Inhalants	20	3	0.4
Heroin	1	⟨ 0.5	0.0
Stimulants	23	6	0.3
Sedatives	10	2	0.1
Tranquilizers	11	2	0.0

Adapted from Johnson LD, O'Malley PM, Bachman JG: *Drug Use by High School Seniors—Class of 1986,* US Department of Health and Human Services publication No.(ADM)87-1535. Rockville, MD, 1987

Because the use of intoxicants is so common among adolescents, the temptation to regard this behavior as normative, and hence acceptable, must be avoided. Accidents are the leading cause of death among adolescents. Of the 25,000 accidental deaths among youth annually, approximately 40%, or 10,000, are alcohol related. Homicide is the second leading cause of death among adolescents. Of the 5,500 adolescent homicide victims each year, 30% are intoxicated at the time they are killed (Table 3).[2,3,4] Drug use is a leading, if not the leading, cause of death among adolescents.

Table 2
Grade of First Use—Class of 1986

Grade	Drug		
	Alcohol	Marijuana	Cocaine
6th	8%	3%	0.2%
7-8th	22	11	0.6
9th	25	12	2
10th	18	11	4
11th	12	9	5
12th	6	5	5
	91%	51%	17%

Adapted from Johnson LD, O'Malley PM, Bachman JG: *Drug Use by High School Seniors—Class of 1986,* US Department of Health and Human Services publication No.(ADM)87-1535. Rockville, MD, 1987

The use of other psychoactive drugs, though less common, is often marked by significant psychosocial disruption, educational and vocational compromise, and somatic consequences in the adolescent. The pattern of adolescent drug use has changed over past decades and will no doubt continue to evolve. Heroin abuse has declined among adolescents during the past 15 years, although heroin addiction among adolescents does still occur. In contrast, cocaine abuse by young people has doubled in the past decade. Seventeen percent of high school seniors report having used this drug at least once, with 5% using in the past month. The use of inhalants, stimulants, tranquilizers, and hallucinogens is additive to a milieu that exposes all adolescents to the risks of drug abuse (Table 1). The pattern of use changes; risk remains a constant. For most young people, such risk arises through their own drug use; nonetheless, even that minority of youth who abstain from psychoactive drugs are not immune to the dangers created by their peers. These young people should not be deprived of our counsel and support as they attempt to maintain their lifestyle in an environment where drug use is the mode.

Table 3
Adolescent Mortality—Ages 15-24
$(n = 38 \text{ million})$[2,4]

CAUSE OF DEATH	RATE PER 100,000	ABSOLUTE NUMBER	PERCENT THAT ARE ALCOHOL-RELATED
ACCIDENTS*	60	25,000	40
HOMICIDE	13	5,500	30
SUICIDE	12.5	5,000	20
MALIGNANCY	6.5	2,400	0
*AUTOMOTIVE	35	15,000	45

THE GUIDE

There is no recipe for the successful management of adolescent drug abuse. No formula or set of formulas would fit the style of all physicians, the characteristics of all families, the problems of all teenagers, or the circumstances of all communities. This guide is not a cookbook but rather a collection of essays and information representing the experience, perspective, and insights of professionals whose careers have been closely associated with the problem of youthful substance abuse.

The content and sequence of chapters were designed to allow the reader either to select an individual chapter of interest that would stand as an independent treatment of a topic, or to progress through the chapters in order, from an understanding of risk factors, through evaluation, to treatment, and to referral. The concluding chapters, **Prevention Programs, Ethical and Legal Considerations, and Specific Drugs,** serve as background for the development of the knowledge base necessary for effective intervention.

Risk Factors and Their Implications for Preventive Interventions for the Physician outlines those circumstances that might make it more likely that a young person would experience drug-related difficulties. The chapter alerts the practitioner to family and environmental issues that require special attention not only during adolescence but also during the years of childhood development that provide the foundation for adolescent behavior. Information on risk factors is presented with the understanding that all young people are in some jeopardy of drug-abuse behavior and that the absence of a specific risk factor in a particular patient does not justify a lack of attention to this issue. **The Role of the Primary Care Practitioner** outlines the breadth of physician responsibilities in the prevention, management, and treatment of adolescent substance abuse and includes guidance as to methodologies for meeting those responsibilities. **Evaluation by Interview** stresses the critical importance of historical information in detecting and assessing drug-abuse behavior and provides practical suggestions for effective questioning of the adolescent and the family. **Use of the Laboratory** explains currently available technology for the detection of drugs of abuse in body fluids, with attention to the applicability, limitations, and cost of each methodology. The chapter on **Referral** provides information on treatment modalities for drug-abusing adolescents, preparing the teenager and the family for referral, and the role of the primary care practitioner after a referral has been made.

Prevention Programs presents an historical perspective regarding initiatives designed to preclude or delay drug abuse behavior or to minimize its consequences. Information on the efficacy of those initiatives is provided when evaluative data are available. **Ethical and Legal Considerations** outlines the evolution of the rights of minors to consent to or deny consent for care, the latitude and limitations of confidentiality, and the role of the courts and the law in assisting in the care of the self-destructive young person. An understanding of applicable law and ethics is essential to addressing the often sensitive and complex relationships between drug-abusing young people and their families. The guide concludes with a reference chapter on **Specific Drugs,** which is designed to assist the practitioner in an understanding of the pharmacologic, psychoactive, and somatic consequences of particular drugs of abuse, with references provided for those circumstances when more detailed information may be needed.

Certain philosophies have directed the style, semantics, and content of this guide. First, the challenge of preventing the consequences of drug abuse among children and adolescents is not the exclusive property of any one group of professionals. Not only are all health professionals, parents, educators, lawyers, clergy, and others welcome to join in meeting this challenge, but we also suggest that not to join is to be negligent. Next, the terms "drug use" and "drug abuse" are far more a matter of literary style than of meaning. Any use of a psychoactive drug by a young person has a health implication. Certainly there is a difference between driving an automobile after consuming one beer or a six-pack, but that difference is one of degree. Similarly, the word "normative" is a statistical term that does not translate as "healthy." Exceeding the speed limit on the highway at one time or another may be "normative," but it is not "safe." Alcohol or marijuana use by older adolescents may be "normative," but it is not "healthy." Finally, at times bright, dedicated, and experienced professionals differ sharply in their approaches to youthful drug abuse. Some would strive to create an adolescent society that is drug free. Others would see that goal as unattainable and work toward minimizing the risks of inevitable drug use by teenagers. Such an approach would be regarded by some as tacit approval of risky and illegal behavior. These divergent groups have two things in common. No one knows the right answer, and no one would wish young people harm. In the absence of a known "right answer," the guide attempts to present all approaches. Facts and data are included when they are available. The reader is encouraged to develop his or her own approach and philosophy to the problem of adolescent substance abuse and thereby bring to this challenge the vigor of a thoughtful personal commitment.

REFERENCES

1. Johnson LD, O'Malley PM, Bachman JG: *Drug Use by High School Seniors—The Class of 1986,* US Department of Health and Human Services publication No.(ADM)87-1535. Rockville, MD, 1987
2. Centers for Disease Control: Alcohol and violent death—Erie County, New York, 1973—1983. *MMWR* 1984;33:226-227
3. Centers for Disease Control: Temporal patterns of motor- vehicle-related fatalities associated with young drinking - United States, 1983. *MMWR* 1984;33:699-701
4. Goodman RA, Mercy JA, Loya F, et al: Alcohol use and interpersonal violence: Alcohol detected in homicide victims. *Am J Pub Health* 1986;76:144-149

RISK FACTORS AND THEIR IMPLICATIONS FOR PREVENTIVE INTERVENTIONS FOR THE PHYSICIAN

INTRODUCTION

The evaluation, management, referral, and long-term care of the adolescent who is seriously involved in substance abuse is marked by the difficulty of such work, the time and expense of treatment, and the frequency with which best efforts nevertheless result in a poor outcome. Our foremost goal should be to recognize young people at risk of drug dependence and to intervene before the establishment of patterns of drug-use behavior that will be difficult to alter. Sadly, the initial symptoms of drug use by young people often go unrecognized by physicians who are trained to associate only the later stages of such use with clinical problems. The purpose of this chapter is to define that subgroup of children who appear to be at special risk of developing a drug-abuse problem. Armed with a knowledge of risk factors and an awareness of the prevalence of substance abuse and of the health and social consequences of drug use, the health professional is in an advantageous position not only to prevent the adolescent from becoming more deeply involved in drug abuse but also to intervene before a drug problem even arises.

Physicians who care for children are in a unique position to intervene in the early stages of substance abuse. They have the advantage of a long-term relationship with children, youth, and families. They are familiar with the developmental stages of childhood, the changing relationship between parents and children, and the personality traits that can make a child particularly susceptible to drug use. Since parents often turn to physicians for advice, messages to parents on the harmful effects of tobacco, alcohol, and other drugs should be part of general health promotion initiatives and should be delivered on a routine basis.[1] To be successful in drug-abuse prevention and intervention, the health professional must be knowledgeable about risk factors for substance abuse and must be alert to children and youth who may be at increased risk. Twenty percent of high school seniors smoke cigarettes daily, nearly three million teenagers between the ages of 14 and 17 are estimated to be problem drinkers, and approximately two thirds of American youth try an illicit drug before they finish high school. Given these statistics, it is very likely that any physician caring for youth will encounter patients suffering from the effects of smoking, alcohol abuse, and other drug use.[2] The abuse of alcohol, other drugs, and tobacco continue to be widespread and to have serious public health implications. While some individuals may discontinue the use of these substances after a brief trial period, initial experimentation with tobacco, alcohol, and other drugs leads all too often to dependence.

Initial drug use is, moreover, now occurring at an earlier age. Ten times as many high school seniors report that they began drinking before leaving the sixth grade as did a decade ago.[2] The percentage of students using drugs by the sixth grade has tripled since 1975.[3] In the early 1960s, marijuana use was virtually nonexistent among 13-year-olds; at the present time, one in six 13-year-olds has used marijuana.[3] "Crack," a highly addictive, inexpensive, smokable form of cocaine, is now widely available. Cocaine use among teenagers has increased: 17% of the high school senior class of 1985 reported that they had used cocaine in the past year.[2] The 1986 National Household Survey of Drug Use reveals some potentially serious developments in patterns of drug abuse by 12-17-year-old youth, the youngest age group surveyed. Twenty-four percent of boys and 23% of girls in this age group had used an illicit drug within the last year. Use of both alcohol and cigarettes by persons in this age group also increased between 1982 and 1985. Marijuana use by 12-17-year-olds as a group increased slightly between 1982 and 1985, from 11.5% to 12.2%. The proportion of 12-13-year-olds who had used marijuana increased from 2% to 6%, while the proportion of 14-15-year-olds who had used the drug increased from 8% to 14% during this period. Furthermore, among 12-17-year-olds who have tried marijuana, 23% of boys and 10% of girls have used it more than 100 times.

Patterns of alcohol, tobacco, and marijuana use among youth are of special concern because these three substances are often considered "gateway" drugs.[4] Most people who become seriously involved with illicit drugs have started with these substances.[4,5] For girls, tobacco use seems to be an especially important predictor of subsequent escalation of drug use. Of course, this sequence of drug use is not absolute. In some communities, particularly among children in ethnic minority groups, inhalants may be the gateway drugs. In addition, some adolescents will try a drug only briefly. There is evidence that persons who initiate drug use very early (under age 15) or late (after age 24) tend to develop the most dysfunctional drug-use patterns. Underlying psychiatric problems have been associated with early and late onset of drug use.[6] In contrast, most drug use initiated between the ages of 15 and 24, the period of greatest risk for initiation, appears to be related to peer and social influence.

Knowledge of the psychosocial and biological factors that play a role in the abuse of tobacco, alcohol, and other drugs has grown substantially in the last decade. Studies have shown that vulnerability to drug use and abuse is increased in children who have low self-esteem, a feeling of not belonging, a high need for social approval, inadequate bonding to family and society, inadequate communication and coping skills, inability to defer gratification, and inability to accept the consequences of their actions.[7] Relatively few studies have focused on childhood and preadolescent predictors of drug involvement. Most have focused on adolescents. Multiple factors appear to predispose adolescents to drug-use problems. The interplay of genetic influences, parental influences, peer group pressures, and sociocultural influences and values is important. These various risk factors probably interact with the individual's own personality to determine whether he or she will develop chemical dependence.

Research has shown that some children are at greater risk of becoming seriously involved with alcohol and drugs than others. Although a multitude of risk factors have been associated with adolescent drug abuse, for the sake of clarity of discussion these characteristics have been grouped into four classifications: family history of alcoholism or drug abuse; other family factors; peer factors; and individual characteristics and psychopathology. Characteristics that should alert the physician to the possibility that a certain patient is at high risk include the following.

Family History of Alcoholism or Drug Abuse

Children of substance abusers are one of the populations at highest risk for substance abuse and other problem behaviors. Both genetic factors and family role models are often involved in predisposing individuals to alcohol abuse. Vulnerability to alcoholism has been well established.[8] The results of family, adoption, and twin studies suggest that both genetic and environmental factors are involved in its etiology. For example, family studies have shown that alcoholism tends to run in families, which may be explained by both genetic and environmental influences. The role of genetic factors in alcoholism has been strongly suggested by results of adoption studies that have found that male adoptees with at least one alcoholic biological parent are three to four times more likely to abuse alcohol than adoptees with biological parents who did not abuse alcohol. Twin studies in which monozygotic twins show higher concordance for alcohol abuse than dizygotic twins also demonstrate the influence of genetic factors. Children of alcoholics are four to five times more likely to become alcoholics than are other children.[9] Evidence indicates that there may be biologically measurable differences in children of alcoholics that may be related to susceptibility to alcoholism.[10]

Other Family Factors

Another family factor that has been shown to increase the likelihood of initiating alcohol or drug experimentation is coming from a home in which parents, older siblings, or other family members smoke, drink, or use drugs. Parental drug use or condonation of drug use also increases the likelihood of drug abuse among children.[11] Parents, in summary, serve as models for their children. Children whose parents smoke, drink, or abuse drugs are more likely to do so than those whose parents do not. Parents who express favorable attitudes toward drug use increase their children's likelihood of abusing these substances. Attitudes and beliefs developed early in childhood concerning the self-administration of medicines and abusable substances may predispose children toward use of substances later in life. Parental attitudes and behaviors regarding the use of substances in the home—such as involving the child in lighting cigarettes, serving drinks, and taking medications without supervision—may influence the development of attitudes and beliefs favorable to drugs and alcohol.[12]

Three parental factors help to predict the child's initiation into drug use: the parents' drug-using behaviors, parental attitudes about drugs, and parent-child interactions.[13] Inconsistent parental discipline and excessive permissiveness or, conversely, severe parental discipline and little praise, have all been found to be associated with higher rates of substance abuse. Positive family relationships and attachment appear to discourage adolescents' initiation into drug use. Children whose parents provide authoritative discipline involving warmth and a willingness to discuss the rationale and consequences of behavior tend to abstain from drug use.[5]

Children from families in which other close family members have a history of criminal or antisocial behavior are more likely to abuse drugs than children whose relatives have not been involved in such behavior.[5]

Finally, children from disadvantaged and socially isolated families, including many minority children, would also appear to be at increased risk for chemical dependency.

Peer Factors

Children whose friends, siblings, or both, use alcohol and other drugs are much more likely to use them than those whose peers do not. Having friends who are drug users is among the strongest predictors of drug use; moreover, there is good evidence that friends rather than strangers generally initiate the young person into drug use. Having friends who regularly drink, smoke, or use other drugs places the preadolescent at high risk for drug use. By the teenage years, peer influence may have become, to some degree, a neutral factor through the natural process of selecting peers like one's self and one's family.

Children at highest risk for substance abuse may be those who are mobile and must enter new school and social systems. Those peer groups most open to the new arrivals are most likely the same groups most willing to take risks—risks with new behaviors, sex, and drugs. Another factor affecting peer selection is rejection of family values, which frequently is associated with another risk factor for drug abuse mentioned earlier, namely, styles of parental discipline.

Individual Characteristics and Psychopathology

Differences in the values, attitudes, and aspirations of young people also influence their risk of drug abuse. A desire for independence based on achievement is one of the strongest factors to protect a young person from drug abuse and to encourage the individual to cease drug use after experimentation. Youth who are aware of and knowledgeable about the medical, social, and legal consequences of drug abuse and who care about their health and future tend to be less likely to experiment with drugs. Adolescents who are not interested in school and academic achievement are, on the other hand, more likely to use drugs. Children who fail in school for whatever reason—lack of ability, boredom, behavioral problems, or learning difficulties—are more likely to experiment with drugs earlier and to become regular users than those who do not fail.[5]

Antisocial behavior, strong rebellious feelings; alienation; lack of strong bonds to family, school, church, and other conventional social institutions; lack of a sense of direction; and low self-esteem have all been shown to increase susceptibility to drug use and abuse. The evidence of a positive correlation between childhood antisocial behavior and subsequent drug abuse is relatively consistent. Early antisocial behavior has been found to predict adolescent substance abuse.[14] A study of urban black first-grade male students found a positive correlation between aggressiveness—especially when accompanied by shyness—and substance use ten years later.[15]

Use of certain drugs by some adolescents may represent an attempt to cope with psychological distress. An interesting finding in a recent analysis of data on 18-30-year-

olds from the National Institute of Mental Health Epidemiological Catchment Area Program suggests that
having a major depressive episode or anxiety disorder
doubles the risk for later drug abuse/dependence with an
odds ratio of 2.2 for males and 1.9 for females.[16] Other research has established a link between affective disturbance and substance abuse.[17] Both of these studies
suggest an opportunity for identifying high-risk individuals.

CONCLUSION

The health professional who cares for children and youth
can play a critical role in the prevention of substance abuse
and in the early intervention with those patients who have
already begun to use drugs.[18] Prerequisites to successful
drug-abuse prevention are a knowledge of those factors
that place a young person at special risk, a sensitivity to
the early signs of drug abuse, and an awareness of the high
prevalence of drug use by young people. The physician's
longstanding relationship with children and families and
understanding of normal development allow him or her to
appreciate both deviations from the normal and emerging
risks for deviance. The potential to intervene before problems arise or at the first signs of difficulty is both the opportunity and obligation of those who care for youth.

REFERENCES

1. Macdonald DI: Drugs, smoking and adolescence. *Am J Dis Child*
    1984;138:117-125
2. Johnson LD, O'Malley PM, Bachman JG: *Drug Use by High School
    Seniors - The Class of 1986,* US Department of Health and Human
    Services publication No. (ADM)87-1535. Rockville, MD, 1987
3. Miller JD, Cisen IH, Abelson HI: *National Survey on Drug Abuse:
    Main Findings,* 1982. National Institute on Drug Abuse, (ADM)83-
    1263, Rockville, MD, 1983
4. Kandel DB: *Longitudinal Research on Drug Use: Empirical Find-
    ings and Methodological Issues.* New York, John Wiley & Sons,
    1978

5. Hawkins JD, Lishner DM, Catalano LF: Childhood predictors and the prevention of adolescent substance abuse, in Jones CL, Battjes RJ (eds): *Etiology of Drug Abuse: Implications for Prevention,* US Department of Health and Human Services publication No.(ADM)85-1335. Government Printing Office, 1985

6. Robbins LN, Przybeck TR: Age of onset of drug use as a factor in drug and other disorders, in Jones CL, Battjes RJ (eds): *Etiology of Drug Abuse: Implications for Prevention,* US Department of Health and Human Services publication No.(ADM)85-1335. Government Printing Office, 1985

7. Hawkins JD, Lishner DM, Catalano LF, Howard MD: Childhood predictors of adolescent substance abuse: Towards an empirically grounded theory. *J Children in Contemporary Society* 1986; 18:1-65

8. Cloniger CR: Genetic and environmental factors in the development of alcoholism. *Psychiatr Treat Eval* 1983;5:487-496

9. Macdonald DI, Blume S: Children of alcoholics. *Am J Dis Child* 1986;140:750-754

10. Schukit MA: Biologic markers: Metabolism and acute reactions to alcohol in sons of alcoholics. *Pharmacol Biochem Behav* 1980;13(suppl 1):9-16

11. McDermott D: The relationship of parental drug use and parents' attitudes concerning adolescent drug use. *Adolescence* 1984;19:89-97

12. Bush PJ, Dannotti RJ: The development of children's health orientations and behaviors: Lessons for substance abuse prevention, in Jones CL, Battjes RJ (eds): *Etiology of Drug Abuse: Implications for Prevention,* US Department of Health and Human Services publication No. (ADM)85-1335. Government Printing Office, 1985

13. Kandel DB, Logan JA: Patterns of drug use from adolescence to young adulthood: Periods of risk for initiation. continued use and discontinuation. *Am J Pub Health* 1984;74:660-666

14. Johnson BB, O'Malley PM, et al: Drugs and delinquency: A search from causal connections in longitudinal research on drug use, in Kandel DB(ed): Washington, DC, Hemisphere-Wiley, 1978

15. Kellam, SG, Simon MC: Mental health in first grade and teenage drug, alcohol and cigarette use. *J Drug Alcohol Dependence* 1980;5:273-304

16. Christie KA, Burke JD, Regier DA, Rae DS, Boyd JH, Locke BZ: Epidemiologic evidence for early onset of mental disorders and increased risk of drug abuse in young adults. *Am J Psychiatry* (in press)

17. Kandel DB, Davies M: Adult sequelae of adolescent depressive symptoms. *Arch Gen Psychiatry* 1986;23:255-261

18. Macdonald DI: Prevention of adolescent smoking and drug use. *Pediatr Clin North Am* 1986;33:(3)995-1005

Chapter 2

ROLE OF THE PRIMARY CARE PRACTITIONER

Although most primary care physicians have not been trained in the area of substance abuse, their relationship with the child/adolescent, rapport with the family, and position in the community clearly give them the opportunity to play a crucial role in the prevention, management, and treatment of adolescent substance abuse.

The primary care physician has a key role in seven areas: 1) anticipatory guidance; 2) recognition of drug use and abuse; 3) treatment; 4) referral; 5) family support; 6) education; and 7) community action.

ANTICIPATORY GUIDANCE

The practice of anticipatory guidance, that is, providing counsel regarding potential problems, is a constant theme in providing care for the young. It begins with the first prenatal visit and extends through well-baby check-ups. This same concept of health maintenance applies throughout childhood and adolescence, and key developmental issues should be addressed at specific critical stages. Hence, education of the individual about tobacco, alcohol, and drug use should begin in childhood when family standards and values in general are being assimilated.

Well-child visits during the prepubertal or school years provide many opportunities to discuss drug use with the child (Table 1). One may ask a youngster if these topics are being discussed in school, and if so, in what classes. The physician may ask, "Tell me what you've learned about drugs (cigarettes, or alcohol) in school." Another possibility may be to ask if drugs are discussed among friends. The physician may ask whether the child understands what is meant by the terms tobacco, alcohol, and drugs. The physician may also ask if the child has ever wondered why some people use drugs. Does he/she know if drugs are harmful? Does he/she think there is any harm in trying drugs? By opening this dialogue, the physician gives a clear message that drugs and alcohol are not taboo subjects and that they may be discussed at any time. This also gives the physician the opportunity to educate the youngster about taking drugs, being offered drugs, or being forced to use drugs. Children should know that they should tell their parents or another responsible adult as soon as possible if this occurs.

Anticipatory guidance should also include the parents. At a prepubertal visit, the physician should inform the parents that drug use/abuse begins in grade school in some communities.[1] The parents should be encouraged to examine their own beliefs and practices concerning drugs and alcohol and should be reminded that these practices and beliefs influence their child. Parents should be encouraged to discuss drug and alcohol use with their children, even at the grade-school level. Parents should be reminded that children readily perceive inconsistencies between preaching and practice by adults. In some instances, for example, parents may state that they are opposed to their children drinking at parties, yet they use alcohol freely at their own adult parties at home. Their children may think drinking alcohol is one way to be grown up! As another example, children who are warned about taking drugs or pills from strangers may witness a family member who must take a daily prescribed medication. The parent should make sure the child understands the difference between taking a tablet for medication and taking a pill as a street drug.

Anticipatory guidance should continue throughout adolescence. Although large numbers of teenagers have used drugs,[2] some have not, particularly in early adolescence. These youngsters should continue to receive developmentally appropriate information about drugs and alcohol. Anticipatory guidance concerning drug use is not a one-time effort; it should occur at every visit. Both children and adolescents should be encouraged to discuss these issues with their primary care physician.

Table 1
Questions Concerning Drugs for the School-aged Child

Have your teachers ever talked about drugs at school?

What have you learned about drugs at school?

Have you and your friends ever talked about drugs?

Do you understand the word "drugs"? What does it mean?

Have you ever wondered why some people use drugs?

Why do you think grown-ups say that drugs are harmful?

Has anyone ever tried to sell you drugs or tried to force you to take drugs?

RECOGNITION OF DRUG USE AND ABUSE

Patterns of drug use during adolescence have changed over the last few decades[3] and may vary by racial or cultural group.[4] These changing patterns may also affect the manner in which young people who are using drugs come to medical attention. Ten or fifteen years ago, drug dependence in an adolescent was most often recognized in conjunction with an emergency room visit caused by the medical sequelae of drug abuse. With the decreasing use of substances that cause serious illness or major physiologic disturbance and the rising popularity of alcohol and marijuana, it is now less likely that the drug-using adolescent will present for care because of the medical consequences of drug use. Trauma that is secondary to accidental injury while intoxicated would be an exception to this trend. The young person who is using substances will usually come to medical attention for routine health care, for an illness that is unrelated to drug usage, or for a behavioral consequence of drug use such as school failure or delinquency.[5]

It is also important that the physician realize that drug-related problems do not start out as drug addiction. Addiction is the result of a gradual process. There are many ways to stage drug use. One commonly accepted system recognizes five steps:[6]

Stage 0:   Vulnerable youth who are curious about drug use.

Stage 1:   Young people who are learning about the use of drugs to alter their moods.

Stage 2:   Young people who seek the effects of using drugs and acquire their own supply.

Stage 3:   Youth who are preoccupied with moodswings and are addicted to abusing substances.

Stage 4:   Youth who are in the end stage of drug addiction, which is sometimes referred to as the "burnout" stage.

The physician must realize that all adolescents are at risk for drug abuse and should therefore be concerned about drug use or exposure in all adolescents. The adolescent at risk of drug use is the one in the physician's waiting room.

Routine Inquiries

Inquiries about drug use should be a routine part of the evaluation of every adolescent, regardless of the underlying condition or concern that brought the patient to the physician's office.[7] Inquiries concerning drug use are a natural component of evaluation of the usual spheres of psychosocial function such as school performance, family relationships, peer relationships, career plans, and sexual attitudes and practices. To obtain reliable information on drug use, the physician must gather the information in an appropriate setting and use appropriate interviewing skills.[8] Information on drug use (as well as sexual information) should be obtained in privacy. It is unreasonable to expect that a teenager will be truthful regarding sexual practices or drug behavior when the answers must be given in the presence of authority figures or parents. The teenager must expect some confidentiality if candid responses are desired.

There are various approaches to asking appropriate questions concerning drug-use practices of the adolescent patient (see Table 2; also Chapter 3).

Table 2
Sample Questions Concerning Drug Use for Adolescents

I know that many schools have drug problems. Does your school have such a problem?

Do most of your friends drink alcohol or smoke marijuana at parties?

Do any of your friends use drugs other than alcohol or marijuana?

Where do most young people obtain drugs?

Do you smoke cigarettes? How many per day?

Have you ever tried alcohol? Marijuana? Other drugs?

Have you ever been ill as a result of using drugs or drinking? In what way?

Have you ever been in trouble with the law as a result of drugs or alcohol?

Do your parents know that you've used alcohol or _____? What would (did) they say?

Have you ever worried about your alcohol or _____ use?

Have you ever been drunk or stoned and driven a car (or motorcycle)?

While it is certainly possible to ask adolescents directly whether they are using drugs, such an approach may not be effective, for the adolescent may be wary of responding affirmatively. Hence, it is probably best to initiate such questions around the adolescent's environment. Most adolescents will not be afraid to respond to questions about drug use by their peers. After finding out what the adolescent's peer group is doing concerning drugs, the physician may then inquire whether the same practices hold true for this particular adolescent. The physician should determine which drugs are being used, in what settings they are being used, how often they are used, and where they are being obtained. If these questions are presented in a nonjudgmental and sincere manner, the teenager is likely to respond honestly.

The reaction of the primary care physician to the adolescent's answers will in large part determine the validity of future responses. If information regarding drug use by the peer group evokes disgust, dismay, or disapproval from the physician, it is unlikely that further questions will be of any value. If information can be received without conveying dismay, alarm, or condescension, it is likely that the teenager will be truthful when queried about his or her own drug-use behavior. It is quite possible that the adolescent is eager to have a knowledgeable adult with whom to discuss drug use. The primary care physician is in an ideal position to be such an individual.

If the physician elicits a positive drug history from an adolescent (including types of drugs used, frequency of use, the setting of use, and severity of use), he/she must then determine whether drug use is interfering with the adolescent's life. Hence, information about other aspects of psychosocial behavior must be correlated with drug-use practices. For example, it is important to determine how the adolescent is doing in school. Have absences or truancy increased? Have grades deteriorated? If the adolescent is employed, is he/she performing satisfactorily? Has the adolescent ever been arrested or incarcerated, or is there any other evidence of delinquent behavior? Does the adolescent have friends? What do they do for fun? How does the adolescent relate to his/her family? Are there duties at home for which he/she is responsible? Is the adolescent sexually active? Promiscuous? Is the adolescent using sex to obtain drugs? Is there evidence of depression? Is there any evidence of psychopathology for which drugs are being used as an escape? The answers to these questions will help determine if a drug problem exists and clarify areas of dysfunction. They may provide evidence to motivate a troubled adolescent to seek help. An adolescent who is heavily involved with drugs (even alcohol or marijuana) virtually always has other areas of dysfunction—in school, with family, or with peers.

Obtaining the answers to these questions is time-consuming. Primary care physicians should be aware that adolescent visits may require more time than appointments with younger children. They should charge appropriately for the extra time required for provision of optimal health care to this age group.

The answers to the questions outlined will determine the role that the physician will assume with the adolescent. If an adolescent is not using drugs, he/she should be commended and encouraged to continue avoiding them. Adolescents who use alcohol or marijuana only occasionally and who do not show evidence of disruptive behavior should be alerted to areas of potential risk, particularly automobile accidents. If the adolescent is old enough to drive or date, the physician should suggest that the adolescent consider what to do if he/she ever became intoxicated away from home or were a passenger in a car to be driven by someone who is intoxicated. Current national efforts to curb such activity should be brought to the adolescent's attention; these include Students Against Driving Drunk (SADD), Safe Rides, and other similar efforts.

Adolescents at Risk for Drug Use/Abuse

Although the physician should be alert to the possibility of drug use by all adolescents, clearly all adolescents will not have a drug-abuse problem. Some subgroups are at higher risk than others.[9] The strongest predictor of teenage drug use is association with friends who use drugs regularly (see Chapter 1). One must also be aware that drug use is starting at increasingly younger ages. Other risk factors for drug use include low self-esteem and failure to belong to a peer group.[10] Such adolescents are lonely and may find themselves turning to drugs to gain prestige in the eyes of their peers. Indeed, some adolescents may begin to use drugs because they are afraid to "say no" because of peer pressure. The party at which a marijuana "joint" is passed from one young person to another is not uncommon, and the individual who chooses to smoke that joint instead of refusing it may be the one who is afraid to stand up for himself/herself and needs the approval of peers. Improving a child's self-esteem is crucial in helping him/her avoid drugs as well as other unfortunate activities such as premature sexual behavior. Adolescents who are depressed may use drugs to alter their moods; in this case, depression is the major problem. Those who are involved in drugs may also use alcohol and tobacco, engage in premature sexual behavior, and have a history of delinquency. In such cases, alcohol and drug use are only part of the problem.

The Pregnant Teenager

There are approximately 500,000 births to teenagers each year in the United States. Some of these young women use drugs and alcohol. A history of tobacco, alcohol, and drug use should be elicited from every pregnant teenager, and those who use such substances should be informed of the potential consequences to their offspring (see Chapter 8). Many adolescents who seem unconcerned about the effect of drugs upon their own health will respond to counseling when warned about potential ill effects upon the unborn infant.

TREATMENT OPPORTUNITIES

Not all young people who are abusing drugs will require referral for drug treatment. On the contrary, many acute consequences of drug abuse can be, and at times must be, treated without referral or the opportunity for consultation. In addition, as the vast majority of adolescents will at some time use alcohol or marijuana, most adolescent drug use must be addressed by the primary care practitioner (see Chapter 5).

The drug-abusing teenager may first come to medical attention as a result of trauma related to intoxication or secondary to an acute drug overdose. The responsibility of the primary care practitioner is not only to treat the trauma or acute physiologic compromise but also to recognize and assess the extent to which drug abuse, episodic or chronic, has led to the circumstance that mandated medical attention. Such recognition and assessment is a prerequisite to a determination of the need for either office counseling or referral for treatment. Other examples in which the willingness and ability of the primary care practitioner to address an acute situation may lead to continuing treatment for substance abuse include the adolescent who presents for care for an addictive problem or a drug-related illness such as cellulitis or hepatitis. In addition, suicidal and depressed teenagers frequently have drug abuse problems. The skills of the practitioner in treating the presenting complaint will influence subsequent success in addressing underlying issues of substance abuse.

REFERRAL FOR TREATMENT

The responsibility of the primary care physician is not limited to recognizing which teenagers are using drugs. The physician must also determine which adolescents are in trouble because of drugs and how they can be convinced to seek help. Although any drug use by a teenager has potential untoward consequences, not all drug use by adolescents is pathological,[11] nor does all drug use require referral for drug rehabilitation. Many adolescents, however, do need assistance.

Most adolescents have three psychosocial spheres of interaction: school, family, and peers. Adolescents who are having difficulty in any one of those three spheres probably need referral for treatment. The adolescent whose life is disrupted as a result of drug use needs referral for treatment. The adolescent who has had a near tragedy such as an overdose or serious accident needs referral for treatment. The adolescent whose drug overdose may in any way be associated with a suicide attempt needs a referral.

Convincing an adolescent and his/her family that a referral is needed may not be easy. There may be an element of denial concerning drug-use problems or a rejection of conventional values concerning drug use. Some young people may adopt an arrogant or abusive attitude toward the physician who suggests that treatment is needed. In order to facilitate entry of the drug-using adolescent into a treatment program, the primary care physician must avoid taking a critical, judgmental, or adversarial role. Coercion is indicated in life-threatening situations; however, it should be reserved for patients who have not responded to more positive approaches. The physician may find that the adolescent will accept the referral if treatment is directed towards one area that is giving him/her difficulties, such as school. The physician may note, "Charles, you used to be an A student in grade school. Your grades have dropped, teachers are sending you poor report cards, and your family is concerned. I think you may need help to keep up your scholastic achievement." Compassionate concern is the physician's best tool in helping a youngster accept referral for treatment.

Most primary care physicians, including specialists in adolescent medicine, have not been trained in drug treatment. Successful treatment of the addicted adolescent or the frequent user often requires a multidisciplinary team

Table 3
Criteria for Treatment and Referral of the Adolescent Substance Abuser*

FOLLOW-UP CARE BY PRIMARY CARE PHYSICIAN

Physician/family practitioner knowledgeable in these areas

Drug use intermittent, experimental, and not unusual for age/sociocultural group

No significant psychopathology

Function in educational, social, or vocational sphere unimpaired

Reasonable progress in developmental tasks

No antisocial behavior

REFERRAL TO SPECIALIZED PRACTITIONER

Lack of experience or uncertainty on part of the primary physician

Significant drug abuse (frequent/regular, major life concern)

Psychopathology requiring evaluation and care

Impaired function in educational, social, legal, or vocational sphere

In certain instances (i.e., when a specialized unit is available) evaluate on an inpatient basis.

REFERRAL TO INPATIENT DRUG TREATMENT PROGRAM

Compulsive drug abuse

Impaired function in educational, social, legal, or vocational sphere

Imminent danger to physical or mental health of patient

Persistent antisocial behavior

Failure of outpatient treatment

Psychopathology requiring behavior control, medication, or both

* Adapted from Millman RB: Treatment and modalities, in Litt IF (ed): **Adolescent Substance Abuse, Report of the l4th Ross Roundtable on Critical Approaches to Common Pediatric Problems.** Columbus, OH, Ross Laboratories, I983, pp. 63-64

whose members are familiar and experienced with both substance abuse and the adolescent age group (Table 3). Effective therapy cannot be expected while an adolescent is still abusing drugs: this behavior must be curtailed. Various treatment modalities have been developed, some of which are more effective than others. These include both outpatient and residential treatment programs[12] (see Chapter 5). All physicians should become familiar with the treatment programs available in their communities and develop a relationship with at least one such facility so that referral can be made on a regular basis. Unfortunately, treatment facilities are limited in many communities, particularly for children from poor families.

After referral, the primary care physician should maintain contact with the adolescent and family. This not only continues to educate the physician concerning drug-use and drug-referral programs but also gives the distinct message that the primary care physician cares about the patient even if he/she disapproves of the adolescent's drug practices.

RESPONSIBILITY TO THE FAMILY

The primary care physician who cares for adolescents also has a responsibility to the family. There are at least three issues that the primary care physician must face with respect to the family and the adolescent drug user: 1) confidentiality; 2) the family problem; and 3) intervention and prevention.

Confidentiality

In order to obtain a reliable drug history, the physician must assure the adolescent patient of confidentiality. This confidentiality must be respected unless the adolescent's life or that of another person is at stake. One could argue that any alcohol or drug use by an adolescent automatically means his/her life or someone else's life may be at stake. That is a judgment that each clinician must make based on the information presented. The adolescent who is dependent upon drugs is obviously in danger. Decisions concerning confidentiality are more difficult when the adolescent is engaged in frequent recreational use of drugs. If the physician reveals the recreational drug use to the patient's parents, he or she runs the risk of losing the patient's confidence and hence being unable to maintain rapport with the adolescent and to make a referral if necessary. The patient's behavior at home and at school may help the clinician in this difficult decision. Keeping drug use confidential from the family is not a goal in itself, and indeed most families are aware of the adolescent's drug and/or alcohol use. One way to resolve the issue is to interview parents and ask them if they have any concerns about the adolescent's behavior that they wish to discuss. One can preface that statement by saying, "It is difficult to raise adolescents these days. Most parents have concerns in many areas such as school performance, peer groups, dating, sexuality, drug use, smoking, alcohol, and partying. Do you have any such concerns?" This enables the parent to raise the issue of substance abuse if he/she wishes, and it enables the primary care physician to explore this area without violating the patient's confidentiality. The physician may then go back to the adolescent and say, "Your mother has told me that she is worried about your alcohol (or other drug) use. This is something I would like us to discuss together." A meeting can then be set up with the parents, the teenager, and the physician to discuss any of the areas of mutual concern.

To start such a meeting, the physician may ask the adolescent and parents whether the teenager is going to parties. Since a teenager may not know in advance whether alcohol or drugs may be available at the party, the adolescent and parents should face the potential problems that this situation presents. Clearly this is an area that merits a plan. The parents and the physician would naturally prefer that the teenager not use drugs or alcohol and not associate with friends who do so; however, such an expectation may be unrealistic. At parties, the adolescent may either use alcohol or drugs or be in the presence of persons using them. Afterwards, the adolescent may either drive while under the influence of drugs or alcohol or be a passenger in a car driven by an intoxicated driver. Discussions of such situations provide an ideal means of coming to terms with matters related to substance abuse.

Drug Use as a Family Problem

It is possible, even likely, that the adolescent who is using alcohol or drugs is part of a family whose members also use such substances. This possibility may be explored with the adolescent, with the parents, or with the family as a whole. It must be done in a nonjudgmental, open, sincere, and compassionate manner. Parents with a drinking problem will often do nothing about it until they see the same problem in their offspring. In order to help their child, they may be willing to seek help themselves.

Prevention-Intervention

Families are often afraid to ask for help for an adolescent who is having a substance-abuse problem. They fear that the adolescent may be removed from the home or will run away. Parents must be reminded that they have an obligation to discuss alcohol and drugs with their adolescent offspring. Teenagers should have no doubts about their parents' stand on this issue. Just as a drug-using adolescent may scoff at a physician's concerns about drug use, the same adolescent may scoff at his/her parents. This does not mean, however, that the discussion should be avoided.

Parents may need advice on how to broach this discussion and may need to be forewarned about reactions and responses common to some teenagers. The adolescent may complain, "Why are you so uptight about my drinking when you drink also?" In this case, the adolescent may need to be reminded that it is legal for adults to drink. In fairness to the adolescent, however, the parent should acknowledge that although it is legal for adults to imbibe, even adults who drink to excess need help. The teenager should be reminded that drug use is illegal for both adults and adolescents. To have this conversation with one's children may take courage, particularly in one-parent families. The primary care physician may provide strong moral support for the parent.

If it is determined that a patient needs a referral for drug treatment, the parents will need additional encouragement. Frequent contact by phone and in person may be necessary. Fears concerning sending the adolescent to a residential treatment program may need to be allayed. It is probably best to focus on what the drugs have done to the adolescent rather than the drug use per se. For example, a physician may state, "Mrs. Jones, I know you are worried about Tommy being placed in a residential setting. I know you are worried that he will hate you and resent this therapeutic measure, but I think you know that Tommy used to have lots of friends and now he has no friends. Having no friends is not normal in adolescence. It generally means that something is wrong. The fact that he has withdrawn from all of his friends and former activities and is secluded in his room, using drugs, may be his way of telling us that there is something wrong and he needs help from us." This approach will often give the parent courage to follow through with the referral. In all cases, the physician must neither abandon the family in its hour of need nor presume that because he or she can see clearly what is needed that the family will view the situation in the same manner and will accept all recommendations.

THE PHYSICIAN AS EDUCATOR

The primary care physician is not simply responsible for caring for health problems. He or she is also a health educator. Hence, the physician has a role to play in educating patients and family members concerning the hazards of alcohol and drug use and abuse. This may be accomplished in many ways: one-on-one sessions with patients and families, posters in the waiting room, and/or pamphlets that children, adolescents, and family members may read or take home. The primary care physician also has a role to play in the community as health educator concerning drug and alcohol use (see below). The physician is often viewed as an authority figure, and his/her opinion may be respected more readily than that of others.

THE PHYSICIAN'S ROLE IN THE COMMUNITY

Beyond the traditional role played by physicians in providing direct care to young people and their families is the opportunity to participate in school and community health initiatives. Although such activities may be less personal than a doctor-patient relationship, they offer the unique opportunity to influence the well-being of large numbers of adolescents. In addition, physicians involved in these programs gain from the sharing of perspectives among educators, clergy, government officials, concerned parents, and other health professionals. Pooled knowledge and shared perspectives most often result in a more worthwhile initiative and increased benefits to the young people served. In a complex area such as substance abuse, where education and ethics, legislation and law enforcement, and family values and actions are as important as or more important than medical concerns, community-based health-care intervention is greatly improved through physician involvement.

Advocacy Roles and Opportunities

While there are many opportunities for physicians to assume advocacy roles within their communities, such participation has generally remained at a low level. At times, a first step toward involvement is the identification of individuals or groups who are already addressing issues of substance abuse. These may include the following:

Medical Societies

Most national and regional medical and specialty societies have either substance-abuse committees or youth/adolescent committees. Whether dedicated specifically to substance abuse or to a broader range of adolescent health problems, these groups may provide a variety of opportunities for involvement. Included within their activities may be educational programs for physicians or the public, consultation to other community agencies, local legislative action, and opportunities to influence the policies and practices of the national parent organization. It is rare indeed that such committees would not welcome the participation of yet another interested physician.

Local Schools

Perhaps the widest range of opportunities for physician involvement exists in participation in school-related activities. Local school boards often welcome assistance in the formulation of drug-abuse policies and curricula. Meetings of the school board provide a forum for expressing concern and offering direction. Beyond such informal opportunities, it is not uncommon for physicians to be appointed to school committees addressing either drug-abuse curricula or policy issues. At times, state law mandates physician representation on such committees.

Local parent-teacher organizations have by and large maintained an active posture regarding issues related to adolescent substance abuse. Their activities have included educational programs for parents and students as well as initiatives designed to prevent or delay drug use or to minimize the consequences of such use.

Local Governments

Most localities have created committees or agencies to address issues of substance abuse. Often the statute that created these agencies requires physician membership. The structure, function, and name of such agencies may differ. At times, these agencies are purely advisory in nature; however, in many cases, they either control the expenditure of governmental funds or receive funding with which to initiate programs and projects.

Citizen-Parent Action Groups

Particular to the area of adolescent drug-abuse prevention efforts has been the emergence of a multitude of community-based initiatives. Independent of professional or governmental affiliation, such groups usually comprise and are led by concerned parents. These local groups are often part of a national network; however, a variety of independent initiatives may be found in any given locality.

A number of such nonprofessional self-help and advocacy groups have achieved national prominence and are worthy of specific mention. It should be noted that none of these programs has been systematically evaluated, and many advocate somewhat controversial intervention strategies. Mention within this chapter does not imply endorsement of either efficacy or approach.

NATIONAL FEDERATION OF PARENTS FOR DRUG-FREE YOUTH (NFP) is a national umbrella organization of more than 8,000 parent groups and 500,000 members. NFP is primarily involved in public policy promotion and education. The organization's "informed parent groups" provide drug-related education for parents and other interested community members, and they sponsor drug-free youth activities. Among the more popular activities sponsored by NFP and its parent groups are "Project Graduation" and "Safe Homes." Project Graduation provides drug- and alcohol-free activities for graduating high school seniors. Safe Homes encourages parents to pledge drug-free, supervised homes for youth and their friends. National Federation of Parents for Drug-Free Youth, 8730 Georgia Avenue, #200, Silver Spring, MD 20910 (301-585-5437).

PARENT RESOURCES AND INFORMATION FOR DRUG EDUCATION (PRIDE) is primarily an information and referral resource for parents and other interested individuals. PRIDE maintains a comprehensive library of materials related to drug abuse and community action and awareness. PRIDE sponsors conferences and publishes a newsletter. PRIDE, Robert Woodruff Building, Volunteer Service Center, Suite 1012, 100 Edgewood Avenue, N.E., Atlanta, GA 30303 (1-800-241-9746).

MOTHERS AGAINST DRUNK DRIVING (MADD) was established by the mothers of victims of drunk drivers. With membership open to all parents, including fathers, MADD is noted for its efforts in bringing our nation's drunk driving problem to the attention of legislators and the general public. Among the major activities of MADD is the promotion of public policy against drunk driving. The group is also noted for providing victim assistance and community education. MADD has nearly 400 chapters nationwide. MADD, 669 Airport Freeway, Suite 310, Hurst, TX 76053 (817-268-MADD).

TOUGHLOVE is a national network of local self-help programs for families of teenagers troubled by drugs and behavioral problems. Toughlove is a crisis-intervention program that provides support and education for parents seeking to gain the cooperation of and control over their families. Toughlove members practice a distinct, sometimes controversial philosophy that dictates firm (tough) action in exercising parental roles. The program offers a newsletter and educational materials to parent groups. Toughlove, P.O. Box 1069, Doylestown, PA 18901 (215-348-7090).

NATIONAL PARENT-TEACHERS' ASSOCIATION (PTA) is the nation's largest child-advocacy association. PTA has 5.8 million members in more than 25,000 schools. National PTA provides a number of programs through local schools in areas of health, education, and safety. Among their programs in drug and alcohol abuse are the "National Drug- and Alcohol-Abuse Prevention Project" featuring a "Drug- and Alcohol-Awareness Week." "Parenting: The Undeveloped Skill," an education program for parents featuring drug- and alcohol-abuse prevention and general parenting skills, and a number of educational brochures such as "Drug Abuse and Your Teen: What Parents Can Do." National PTA, 700 North Rush Street, Chicago, IL 60611 (312-787-0977).

FAMILIES ANONYMOUS (FA) is a national network of more than 300 local self-help groups patterned after Alcoholics Anonymous. FA groups are open to anyone, including parents, relatives, and friends concerned about drug abuse or related behavioral problems. FA maintains a hotline, helps establish community meetings, and makes referrals to local groups. Families Anonymous, P.O. Box 528, Van Nuys, CA 91408 (818-989-7841).

NARCOTICS ANONYMOUS (NA) is a national network of more than 2,000 regional groups. They are closely patterned after Alcoholics Anonymous (AA). NA groups are conducted by recovered drug addicts, who follow the AA program to aid in rehabilitation. NA publishes a variety of helpful materials for its members, including a directory of group meetings. Narcotics Anonymous, 16155 Wyandotte Street, Van Nuys, CA 91406 (818-780-3951).

ADULT CHILDREN OF ALCOHOLICS (ACOA) is a relatively new network of self-help groups for the children of alcoholics, both young and old. ACOA programs are based on the recognition that family members, especially children, are also victimized by alcoholism, and that the trauma of growing up in an alcoholic family may be lifelong, requiring counseling and support. Adult Children of Alcoholics, P.O. Box 880517, San Francisco, CA 94188 (415-931-2262).

SAFE RIDES is a nationwide program that is frequently affiliated with the Boy Scouts of America. Safe Rides is a loose network of local and regional initiatives that share a common philosophy and function. These programs provide a free and confidential safe ride to any young person who is not in a condition to drive safely or who wants to avoid riding in a vehicle driven by someone who has been drinking or using drugs. Adult involvement in these programs is often limited to an advisory role.

STUDENTS AGAINST DRIVING DRUNK (SADD) is a national organization with some 14,000 chapters in high schools, 4,000 in junior high schools, and 400 in colleges. Specific initiatives include educational programs within schools and the community regarding the dangers of driving while intoxicated, advertising campaigns, and promoting the creation of weekend hot-line services to provide safe rides. Additionally, SADD encourages age-appropriate contacts between teenagers and their parents, and between college students and their schoolmates to facilitate safe behavior if drunkenness were to occur. Students Against Driving Drunk, P.O. Box 800, Marlboro, MA 01752 (617-481-3568).

This sampling of programs provides but a partial listing of the multiple opportunities for involvement that are available to the physician as parent, practitioner, or community leader. Although the efficacy of many of these initiatives remains unproven (see Chapter 6), there is little doubt that the sincere collaboration of a health professional who is willing to learn, teach, and share knowledge and perspective would be of benefit to young people.

CONCLUSION

Although usually not possessing the time, knowledge, or skills to treat the more seriously drug-involved adolescent, the primary care physician can play a critical role in addressing issues of substance abuse among teenagers. Through anticipatory guidance, the emergence of drug abuse problems may be prevented or minimized. Most often the primary care practitioner is the only health professional who is in a position to recognize problems of drug abuse as they evolve and is the clinician most likely to be called to treat the acute consequences of drug use. The longitudinal relationship with the adolescent and the family is an asset not only in the referral process but also in offering support throughout the process of evaluation and treatment. Finally, as an educator and as a facilitator of community action, the primary care practitioner has the opportunity to exert influence upon issues of drug abuse beyond the confines of the practice setting or the individual doctor-patient relationship.

REFERENCES

1. Clayton RR, Ritter C: The epidemiology of alcohol and drug abuse among adolescents. *Adv Alcohol Subst Abuse*, 1985;4:69
2. Johnson LD, O'Malley PM, Bachman JA: *Use of Licit and Illicit Drugs by America's High School Students, 1975—1984,* US Department of Health and Human Services publication No. (ADM) 85-1394. Government Printing Office, 1985
3. Hein K, Cohen MI, Litt IF: Illicit drug use among urban adolescents: A decade in retrospect. *Am J Dis Child*, 1979; 133:38

4. Morgan M, Wingard D, Felice ME: Subcultural differences in alcohol use among youth. *J Adol Health Care,* 1984;5:181
5. Schonberg SK: Diagnosis and recognition of adolescent substance abuse, in Litt IF (ed): *Adolescent Substance Abuse: Report of the Fourteenth Ross Roundtable on Critical Approaches to Common Pediatric Problems.* Columbus, OH, Ross Laboratories, 1983
6. Macdonald DI: *Drugs, Drinking, and Adolescents.* Chicago, Year Book Medical Publishers, 1984
7. American Academy of Pediatrics, Committee on Adolescence: The role of the pediatrician in substance abuse counseling. *Pediatrics,* 1983;72:251
8. Felice ME, Vargish W: Interviewing and evaluation of the adolescent, in Kelly VE (ed): *Practice of Pediatrics.* Hagerstown, MD, Harper & Row, 1984
9. Newcomb MD, Maddahian E, Bentler PM: Risk factors for drug use among adolescents: Concurrent and longitudinal analyses. *Am J Pub Health,* 1986;76:525
10. Kandell DB: Epidemiological and psychosocial perspective on adolescent drug use. *J Am Acad Child Psychiatr,* 1982;21:328
11. Schonberg SK: Perspective on the role of the pediatrician in the management of adolescent drug use. *Pediatr Review,* 1985;7:131
12. Millman RB: Treatment and modalities, in Litt IF (ed): *Adolescent Substance Abuse: Report of the Fourteenth Ross Roundtable on Critical Approaches to Common Pediatric Problems.* Columbus, OH, Ross Laboratories, 1983

Chapter 3

EVALUATION BY INTERVIEW

The primary goal of every clinical encounter with an adolescent is the establishment of a therapeutic alliance. The therapeutic alliance, or working relationship, is necessary for effective communication, which ultimately allows the physician to offer help and the adolescent to accept it. This relationship is especially delicate when substance abuse is a consideration. To achieve this goal, the physician must perceive the adolescent, not the adolescent's parents or other custodians, as the patient. The physician obviously also has a responsibility to the parents or guardians; however, the alliance with the patient must be fundamental. In order to help a young person, the physician must have a genuine interest in the adolescent, have positive feelings about the teenager, attempt to develop trust in the patient, and be capable of empathetic understanding of the adolescent patient's orientation and situation. The physician must accept the role of advocate rather than adversary for his or her young patient.

There are prerequisites for achieving effective clinical working relationships with adolescents. The physician must evidence authenticity or genuineness. The physician who cares for adolescents must be a good listener, be skilled at giving opinions and guidance, yet be able to avoid being judgmental and authoritarian. This does not preclude the physician from having opinions, making judgments, taking positions on issues, and when appropriate, using his or her authority. Integrity and honesty when interacting with the young person and his/her family should be the rule. There may be times when all cannot be shared with the patient or family. The physician must carefully consider the options in such situations before undertaking measures that would jeopardize his or her relationship with the patient, which would not be in the patient's best interest, or would be unethical. Finally, the physician must have the knowledge, skills, and clinical judgment necessary to diagnose and manage the many forms of substance abuse.

Clinical encounters with adolescents who are using illicit drugs and alcohol occur in many different circumstances. The primary care physician's encounter with the substance-abusing adolescent often occurs during the course of a health maintenance, sports, or school examination. In other cases, the office-based physician may be contacted initially by a parent who is concerned about the child's increasingly intolerable behavior. In still others, school or juvenile authorities may encourage the parent to have the young person evaluated for possible substance abuse. Less often, the physician will see a patient in an emergency room following a drug overdose or an untoward effect of a drug or alcohol. Patients seen in this latter circumstance may be approached in a more straightforward fashion, since questions regarding their use of drugs and whether drugs constitute a "problem" have already been answered.

Physicians practicing in hospital outpatient departments or community clinics are more likely than office-based practitioners to have patients referred to them by police, juvenile detention center and half-way house personnel, or by staff members of other community agencies. In such cases, the physician is usually requested by the youth's custodian to document the recent use of drugs or alcohol so that action can be taken against the alleged offender. The physician who accedes to this request should not anticipate an ongoing or helping relationship with the patient. Under these circumstances, it is very unlikely that the adolescent will share any relevant or accurate information that would support a diagnosis of substance abuse. Unless the patient is intoxicated, has used drugs parenterally, or has the rarely present specific physical findings associated with certain drugs, it is impossible to ascertain that the patient has been abusing drugs without the use of laboratory tests.

THE HEALTH MAINTENANCE VISIT

Ideally, the establishment of the working alliance between physician and adolescent should begin during the patient's childhood. Relationships between physician, child, and parents should lay the groundwork for a doctor-adolescent patient relationship that allows confidentiality to develop. The parents in time will realize that a dyad must gradually evolve between doctor and adolescent patient. At a certain time, usually around the ages of 11 to 13 years, the physician should be spending a major part of the visit alone with the patient. As the young person progresses through adolescence, the parents play a less prominent role during the visit. With the adolescent's knowledge, they are, however, informed of important aspects of the visit and are available for consultation with the physician when necessary. The older the adolescent, the more independent of the parents the relationship will become. By middle adolescence, the patient and parents should understand and accept the need for confidentiality. For the most part, what transpires during the visit is between adolescent and physician. The adolescent must realize, however, that the established confidentiality is not unqualified or absolute. Certain information may have to be shared with the parents. Adolescents should be assured that their privacy and integrity will be guarded unless their actions have the potential for or constitute imminent harm to themselves or others. In such instances, the adolescent should have prior knowledge of what will be told to the parents. He/she must be assured that the disclosure will concern only issues threatening his/her immediate welfare and that he or she will have the first opportunity to communicate the information to the parents.

During the preadolescent years, the physician and parents should anticipate and understand the need for future confidentiality. This can be accomplished easily if the necessary groundwork has been done. A conversation with the parents is usually sufficient to set the ground rules for future visits. This gives the parents an opportunity to express their feelings regarding experimentation with drugs and alcohol, sexual activity and contraception, and other important issues. Such a policy establishes guidelines for the physician that may prove helpful if problems eventually do arise.

By early adolescence, the patient should be capable of completing a previsit questionnaire. Such questionnaires are designed to generate a data base specific to the patient and to provide information on a broad variety of clinical issues, including both routine health concerns and matters relating to behaviors such as sexuality and substance abuse. This is an efficient method of data collection for several reasons. Many adolescents, for example, have less trouble sharing "sensitive" information in this way than in face-to-face encounters with the doctor. Table 1 lists examples of the types of questions concerning substance abuse that can be incorporated into a questionnaire. Questions regarding drug use may be used to expand the usual data base sought from all adolescents; they may also be added to the questionnaire when there is reason to suspect that the child is already abusing drugs or is vulnerable to drug abuse.

One may ask additional questions in order to elicit indepth information that may indicate advanced substance abuse (Table 2). These questions should be asked during an interview or physical examination; they are inappropriate for inclusion in a questionnaire. Some adolescents are more likely to give accurate answers when asked the questions during the physical examination. In some respects, they feel less like they are being interrogated, and the questions seem to be more spontaneous and casual. However, other adolescents are more anxious during the physical examination, and this may interfere with data collection. Still others may feel that the physician has detected something on the physical examination that prompted the inquiry. The physician should be alert to these possibilities and modify his or her approach accordingly. The questions in Table 2 are designed to elicit information that might be used as the departure point for a productive dialogue.

Table 1
Questionnaire Items Relevant to Substance Abuse

1. Do you smoke cigarettes?   Y____   N____
2. Do you smoke marijuana?   Y____   N____
3. Do you often feel "bummed out," down,
   or depressed?   Y____   N____
4. Do you ever use drugs or alcohol to
   feel better?   Y____   N____
5. Do you ever use drugs or alcohol when
   you are alone?   Y____   N____
6. Do your friends get drunk or get high at   Y____   N____
   parties?
7. Do you get drunk or get high at parties?   Y____   N____
8. Do your friends ever get drunk or get high
   at rock concerts?   Y____   N____
9. Do you ever get drunk or get high at
   rock concerts?   Y____   N____
10. Have your school grades gone down recently? Y____   N____
11. Have you flunked any subjects recently?   Y____   N____
12. Have you had recent problems with your
    coaches or advisers at school?   Y____   N____
13. Do you feel that friends or parents just do
    not seem to understand you?   Y____   N____

Teenagers seen for routine visits are usually pleasant, articulate, and cooperative. They are aware of the reason for the visit, agree with the need to be in the office, and correctly assume that neither the parent nor the physician has a hidden agenda. Occasionally, the parents will have had a preliminary discussion with the physician and have shared their concern about the possibility of substance use or abuse. The parents should be told that their concern will be presented to the adolescent early in the visit in order to eliminate any element of subterfuge and to preserve the adolescent's trust in the physician. This should be done in a positive, matter-of-fact manner. The physician must project his or her acceptance and understanding of the parental concern and make it clear that the parent was not wrong in sharing the concern with the doctor. It is extremely important that the physician not identify too closely with either the parents or the adolescent. In order to be of help, the physician must maintain the confidence of both the patient and his/her parents and make every effort not to take sides.

Table 2
Open-ended Questions Intended to Provide a Basis for Further Exploration of Advanced Substance Abuse

1. What do your friends do at parties? Do you go to the parties? Do you drink? Get drunk? Get high?

2. Do you drive drunk? Stoned? Have you ridden with a driver who was drunk or stoned? Could you call home and ask for help? What would your parents say? Do?

3. Do you go to rock concerts? Do you drink there? Do you get high? Who drives after the concert?

4. After drinking, have you ever forgotten where you had been or what you had done?

5. Have you recently dropped some of your old friends and started going with a new group?

6. Do you feel that lately you are irritable, "bitchy," or moody?

7. Do you find yourself getting into more frequent arguments with your friends? Brothers and sisters? Parents?

8. Do you have a girlfriend/boyfriend? How is that going? Are you having more fights/arguments with him/her lately? Have you recently broken up?

9. Do you find yourself being physically abusive to others? Your brothers/sisters? Your mother/father?

10. Do you think your drinking/drug use is a problem? Why?

When conducting the interview and taking the history, the physician should consider the patient's age and level of psychosocial maturation. The young person's level of drug and alcohol exposure and experimentation and his/her stage of substance abuse are important factors.

Considerable sensitivity, discretion, tact, and subtlety are required when approaching the subject of substance abuse. The following examples illustrate only a few of the pitfalls that may be encountered. The early adolescent may perceive the physician as being intrusive, or even outrageous, if information is sought in a manner that is too direct or aggressive. As a result, the patient may withhold information or even withdraw completely from the encounter. The middle adolescent may tend to exaggerate his or her responses in order to shock or test the physician. The older adolescent may become defensive or cautious, fearing that answers may be incriminating or may lead to more unwelcome probing. Each adolescent patient is unique, and a uniform or "cookbook" approach is neither possible nor desirable.

Rarely, two extremes of adolescent behavior are encountered; one is a very quiet, noncommunicative teenager; the other, a glib, verbose, and obsequious youngster. Silence on the part of the adolescent does not always indicate uncooperativeness, hostility, or anger; rather, it may signify anxiety about the visit, plain shyness, or inexperience in talking with adults. The talkative and overly cooperative "smoothy" is worrisome. This behavior may reflect a disdain or contempt for authority that, in some cases, may indicate a belief that he/she can get away with anything, including illicit drug and alcohol use. When confronted with such a "charmer," the physician must guard against attempts by the patient to manipulate both the parents and the physician.

Frequently, neither the review of systems nor the physical examination performed as part of a routine health maintenance visit will disclose findings specific to drug abuse. In rare cases, a patient will bear the cutaneous stigmata of intravenous drug abuse, including needle tracks over superficial veins or scars from subcutaneous injection. More often, signs and symptoms secondary to drug abuse such as conjunctivitis from smoking marijuana, constipation due to opiates, or gastritis secondary to excessive ingestion of alcohol, will be erroneously attributed to more common nondrug-related etiologies. The practitioner is most reliant upon an accurate history as an aid in assigning these complaints to their true cause (see Chapter 3).

The value of laboratory testing in screening for drug abuse remains controversial. Periodic urine screening is an accepted component of the ongoing therapy of the known drug abuser; however, routine testing of all adolescents, with or without their knowledge and consent, is not a common practice. Such testing should not be incorporated into the regular care of the adolescent without careful consideration of its potential impact on the relationship between the physician and the adolescent patient. During routine testing of urine or blood, one may occasionally discover proteinuria or eosinophilia, findings that have been associated with opiate abuse. In addition, abnormal liver function enzymes or a false-positive serologic test for syphilis may be indicative of intravenous opiate abuse. Laboratory discovery of an abnormality that reveals previously unsuspected substance abuse is quite rare. Information gathered by interview is far more likely to detect drug abuse than either the physical examination or laboratory findings.

When patients are being seen for health maintenance visits or routine school or sports physical examinations, the physician may attempt to manage early experimentation or early regular use of alcohol or marijuana while preserving confidentiality. Age is a factor; the younger the patient, the more important it is to share information with parents. Experimentation with marijuana by a 13-year-old patient should—in most instances, and with the patient's knowledge—be shared with the parents. Cocaine experimentation by a 17 1/2-year-old young man who requests that his parents not be told may, in certain circumstances, initially be managed by the physician alone. Again, each patient is an individual. Parents vary in their needs and ability to deal with the adolescent. The physician's level of comfort in addressing a given situation will vary. The physician's approach must be matched to the individual patient, the family, and the particular clinical situation.

THE PATIENT SUSPECTED OF OR KNOWN TO BE ABUSING ALCOHOL OR DRUGS

The young patient suspected of, or known to be, abusing substances may be brought to the physician for the express purpose of documenting drug abuse and when indicated, initiating intervention. Such a patient often is forced into a distasteful, adversarial position. The adolescent often does not perceive his/her drug use as a problem, is resentful, and truly believes that the physician's involvement is an intrusion on his/her privacy. The patient may be sullen, belligerent, and at times openly hostile. In such cases, successful intervention requires great skill and patience. Some patients will acknowledge that there is justification for the visit and be relatively cooperative; others, while accepting the need for the visit, will test the physician with provocative posturing and statements. The adolescent must come to realize that the physician can and will deal with the provocations, will be empathetic and understanding, and will maintain control of the clinical encounter. The physician must learn to take the adolescent's "wind out of his sails" and sustain the adolescent's angry barrage of hostile statements and derogatory comments without becoming upset or angry. This is not easy, and there are times when the young patient must be confronted regarding his/her uncooperative and hostile behavior. This confrontation should be accomplished in a cool, matter-of-fact manner using comments such as, "I realize you're angry and certainly don't want to be here, but I wish you would consider my position. I've been asked to do a job and I need your help to do it in the best way I know how." Depending on the teenager's response, the visit may be continued or be terminated in an unemotional and calm manner. A return visit should be arranged. By this time, the patient may have completed his/her testing, accepted the physician as a possible resource, and adopted an improved attitude. Certain patients, on the other hand, may be unable to accept the physician on any terms. If the substance abuse is considered to be a major threat to the patient or his/her family, a referral for specific drug-abuse treatment is warranted. This may have to be accomplished against the patient's will; subterfuge, court order, or even force may be needed.

The physician usually has been provided with some preliminary information by the parents before the initial evaluation. Ideally, a conference with the parents should take place in the office. More often, and realistically, the information is obtained by telephone at the time the appointment is made. It is vital that one or both parents accompany the adolescent to the initial visit. When indicated, the physician may ask that important others, such as a teacher, coach, or school counselor, be present as well. The number of persons invited to the session depends on a number of factors including: 1) the patient's age and level of maturity; 2) the circumstances surrounding the discovery or suspicion of substance abuse; 3) the patient's preference; 4) the availability of others and difficulty of transportation; 5) whether or not the patient has been told the reason for the visit (despite the physician's recommendation that this be done, often it is not, because the parents justifiably fear that the patient will refuse to keep the appointment); and 6) the physician's preference.

The evaluation of the patient suspected of, or known to be, abusing drugs or alcohol should include questions that delve deeper than those asked during a routine or health maintenance visit. These questions may be incorporated into a written questionnaire or integrated into the interview. They should explore the extent of drug and alcohol abuse and related functional disturbance (see Table 3).

Young persons in an advanced stage of substance abuse frequently have a dual diagnosis; the chemical abuse being an associated secondary phenomenon or an attempt by the young person to cope with or assuage the symptoms of a primary emotional problem. Such problems may include depression, character disorders, learning problems, poor impulse control, major thought disorders, and inability to defer gratification, among others. Patients and parents will need to be questioned for evidence of emotional disturbance and personality deterioration. As in other areas of inquiry, the choice between interview and written questionnaire will depend upon the style, judgment, and instincts of the practitioner. Adolescents in advanced stages

---

Table 3.
Questionnaire for Adolescent Patients Suspected of or Known to be Abusing Drugs and/or Alcohol

1. Have you ever been stopped for driving while intoxicated? (drunk/stoned/high?)

2. Have you ever been arrested for possession of drugs, burglary, vandalism, shoplifting, or breaking and entering?

3. Have you ever had to go to an emergency room or doctor's office for a drug-related accident or illness (overdose)?

4. Have you ever overdosed or intentionally tried to kill yourself?

5. Have your grades recently gone down?

6. Did you receive any "Fs" on your last report card?

7. Have you been expelled from school?

8. Have you ever been intoxicated or high (stoned) at school?

9. Have you ever been caught at school for drug or alcohol possession?

10. Have any of your friends been admitted to a drug-treatment center?

11. What drugs, if any, have you used in the past? How much?

12. What drugs, if any, are you currently using? How much?

13. Have you ever experienced "blackouts" while drinking heavily? (For example, have you awoken unable to remember what happened the night before?)

14. Has your alcohol or drug use caused problems with your friends and/or family?

15. Have you ever gotten into trouble at work or at school because of alcohol or drug use?

16. Do you often wake up with a "hangover"?

of substance abuse may often be uncooperative and give incomplete or inaccurate answers. Questions of the parents are intended to identify behaviors associated with advanced stages of substance abuse of which the parent may be unaware and which the patient may be unlikely to disclose (see Table 4).

Table 4
Questionnaire for the Parent(s) of the Adolescent Suspected of or Known to be Abusing Drugs and/or Alcohol

1. Does your daughter/son spend many hours alone in his/her bedroom apparently doing nothing?

2. Does your son/daughter resist talking to you or persistently isolate himself/herself from the family?

3. Has your daughter's/son's taste in music had a dramatic change to hard rock music?

4. Has there been a definite change in your son's/daughter's attitude at school? With his/her friends? At home?

5. Has your daughter/son shown recent pronounced mood swings with increased irritability and angry outbursts?

6. Does your son/daughter always seem to be unhappy and less able to cope with frustration than he/she used to be?

7. Has your daughter's/son's personality changed from being a considerate and caring person to being selfish, unfriendly, and unsympathetic?

8. Does your son/daughter always seem to be confused or "spacey"?

9. Have money or valuable articles recently disappeared from your home?

10. Has your daughter/son begun to neglect household chores and homework?

11. Has there been a change in your son's/daughter's friends from age-appropriate friends to older, "unacceptable" associates?

12. Has there been a change in your daughter's/son's appearance (i.e., sloppy dress and poor grooming and hygiene)?

13. Have there been excuses and alibis made, and has there been lying in order to avoid confrontation or not to get caught?

14. Do you feel you have lost control of your son/daughter?

15. Has your daughter/son begun lying in order to cover up sources of money and possessions?

16. Have there been episodes of "ditching" or "skipping" school? Has your son/daughter lied to cover up bad report cards?

I7. Have there been stealing, shoplifting, or encounters with the police?

I8. Has your daughter/son become a "con artist"?

I9. Have you noticed a marked increase in your son's/daughter's interest in drugs, drug literature, and the drug "culture" (i.e., clothing and accouterments, paraphernalia, belt buckles, and tee shirts with a drug theme)?

20. Has your daughter/son recently quit a sport or dropped out school clubs, social groups, stopped music lessons, quit the band or orchestra, or lost interest in a hobby?

2I. Has there been a deterioration of school performance, frequent truancy, or conflict with coaches or teachers?

22. Do you feel your daughter/son has become untrustworthy, insincere, and distrustful ("paranoid")?

23. Has he/she become unpredictable or rebellious?

24. Has your son/daughter been verbally abusive to you or your spouse?

25. Has your daughter/son been physically abusive to you or your spouse?

26. Has your son/daughter tried to introduce any of your other children to drugs or alcohol?

27. Has your daughter/son talked about suicide or running away?

28. Is your son/daughter more argumentative lately? Does he/she tend to blame others for his/her problems?

29. Is there a paranoid flavor to all of your daughter's/son's relationships with adults, siblings, and authority figures?

When there is a high suspicion of or prior knowledge that the adolescent is abusing drugs, the review of systems and physical examination should be conducted in search of drug related signs and symptoms. Similarly, the laboratory assessment must be more extensive in search of abnormalities resulting from chronic or excessive alcohol or drug abuse and, when appropriate, to identify the types of chemicals being abused. (see Chapters 8 and 4).

At the conclusion of the initial evaluation, the patient should be asked to return within five to seven days. At the return visit, assessment of the young person and the family should continue. The results of laboratory tests should be reviewed with the patient. With the patient's knowledge, and as appropriate, this information should be shared with the parents. The adolescent may resist returning, attempting to ensure the physician that there really is no problem and the substance abuse is nothing that he/she cannot handle. Some patients may resist initially but actually comply if the physician is firm in his/her conviction that intervention is necessary and that a return visit is expected.

The information gathered and rapport established through the interview will serve as the building block upon which subsequent therapeutic initiatives will be constructed. Assessment, counseling, and referral are dependent not only upon obtaining accurate information but also upon the maintenance of a therapeutic alliance between physician, adolescent, and family. Attaining these goals requires thoroughness and tact.

Chapter 4

USE OF THE LABORATORY

PREFACE

Improved methodologies now allow for the detection of drugs of abuse in body fluids with a high degree of accuracy. In part secondary to these recent advances, "drug screening" has become an issue of some controversy. Both legal and ethical issues continue to be subjects of debate in the application of these methodologies to either individual patients or groups of young people. However, there is no question that the physician caring for young people should be familiar with the spectrum of analytic techniques available and the benefits and shortcomings of each. This chapter, reprinted with the permission of the American Medical Association, contains the full text of a 1986 report prepared by their Council on Scientific Affairs (JAMA 1987; 257:3110-3114). The report was written with regard to the technical aspects of drug testing and from the perspective of the utilization of such testing on adults, either within the workplace or in forensic circumstances. The application of routine screening procedures to children and adolescents was neither endorsed nor implied by the AMA report.

Scientific Issues in Drug Testing

Synopsis

Testing for drugs in biologic fluids, especially urine, is a practice that has become widespread. The technology of testing for drugs in urine has greatly improved in recent years. Inexpensive screening techniques are not sufficiently accurate for forensic testing standards, which must be met when a person's employment or reputation may be affected by the results. This is particularly a concern during screening of a population in which the prevalence of drug use is very low, in which the predictive value of a positive result would be quite low. Physicians should be aware that results from drug testing can yield accurate evidence of prior exposure to drugs, but they do not provide information about patterns of drug use, about abuse of or dependence on drugs, or about mental or physical impairments that may result from drug use. (**JAMA** 1987;257:3110-3114)

The technology of screening for drugs in blood and urine has greatly improved in recent years, and it is now possible to determine drug levels in body fluids with a high degree of qualitative and quantitative accuracy. However, the most accurate analytic techniques are often quite expensive and, therefore, are not suitable for large-scale drug screening programs. Less expensive techniques often result in less accuracy, especially when they are not confirmed by more specific techniques.

Laboratory procedures are divided into screening tests and confirming tests. Screening tests are designed for maximum sensitivity, and specificity is often sacrificed. That is, in a screening procedure, it is important to use tests that yield few or no false-negative results, since a negative result terminates the testing process. Confirming tests, on the other hand, are more specific in that they separate true-positive from false-positive results, although some have high sensitivity as well.

Several important issues must be considered in developing a program for testing drugs in urine:

1. **What are the objectives of a testing program?** Is the tester interested in maximizing the likelihood of detecting any use of a wide variety of drugs, or is the tester more concerned with heavy use of a few substances? Is the tester monitoring a "general" population, in which the prevalence of drug use may be relatively low, or a population of known drug users or persons whose known clinical impairment

may be a result of drug use? Will the results be used in a manner that may substantially affect a person's employment or reputation? These objectives must be clearly established before tests with appropriate sensitivities, specificities, and costs can be selected and before administrative policies can be formulated.

The selection of the population for testing is crucial, since the prevalence of drug use varies among populations, and the prevalence greatly affects the positive predictive value of the test, that is, the percentage of true-positive results in all the positive results. For a drug test that has 90% specificity and 99% sensitivity, if the prevalence of use of the drug is 1%, the predictive value is 9%. Thus, if 10,000 people are screened and 100 (1%) use a certain drug, 99 of these 100 would test positive (99% sensitivity) and 990 of the 9900 nonusers would test positive (10% false-positive, or 90% specificity), so that the predictive value would be 99/1089, or 9%. Conversely, 91% of the positive results, on confirmation, would be found to be false. The predictive value increases to 52% at a 10% prevalence.

2. How broad a screen should be performed? Should a procedure test for only one or two substances or for a wide range of compounds? Although a narrow spectrum is less expensive, once the persons to be tested are aware of which drugs are included in the screen, they can switch to other drugs.

3. What is the sensitivity of the screening procedure? Most screening procedures are extremely sensitive and should detect drugs in 99% or more of the specimens in which they are present at concentrations greater than or equal to a predetermined analytic cutoff level. However, specificity may be poor, with false-positive rates in some highly sensitive screening procedures as high as 35%.[1] To confirm the presence of a drug in the urine, it is necessary to use a second procedure,[2] which should be highly specific (99%) for the drug reported in the screening procedure.

4. **What is the specificity of the confirming procedure?** Confirmatory procedures for both limited- and broad-spectrum screening programs can be expensive. Therefore, how the results will be used most often dictates which confirmatory procedures are employed. If results will be used solely for diagnostic purposes or to monitor progress in a rehabilitation program, tests that are often referred to as "clinical confirmatory procedures" may be used. These procedures must be highly reliable but would not be expected to withstand the scrutiny of litigation.

Results that may have an impact on the life, liberty, property, reputation, or employment of the person being tested must be able to withstand the scrutiny of litigation and therefore must meet forensic standards.

Forensic confirmations must (1) unequivocally establish the identity of the compound(s) detected, (2) quantitate the compound(s) detected, and (3) document a chain of custody.[3] The key for a forensic confirmation is to establish objective criteria for testing and reporting and then apply the objective criteria to the laboratory data, reporting as positive only those specimens that fully meet the criteria.[4]

5. **Is there a well-documented chain of custody?** This issue is often overlooked. The urine should be collected under direct visualization to verify the source of the sample. The urine should then be labeled carefully to prevent intentional or inadvertent confusion of the samples. Each time a sample changes hands, an authorized person should sign for the sample and verify that it is in a sealed container. Chain-of-custody forms are designed to establish an audit trail so that a specimen's history can be reconstructed accurately for the court. The procedure is quite simple but requires diligence. The testing laboratory should save a portion of the sample in its original container for future testing should any question arise regarding the results.[5]

6. What do the results of urine testing for drugs mean? Within the limits of accuracy of the tests that are used and the administrative security of the program in which these tests are carried out, drug testing only differentiates between persons who have exposed themselves to the drugs being tested for and those who have not. The results do not give any indication of the pattern of drug use (method of administration, frequency of use, time of last use, or amount used), of whether the individual abuses or is dependent on a drug, or of whether an individual is impaired physically or mentally by the use of the drug. A possible exception to the latter limitation is testing of urinary ethyl alcohol, whose concentrations often can be correlated with blood alcohol concentrations, from which a degree of impairment may be determined.[6-10] For virtually all other drugs, the assignment of impairment from a single urine drug analysis is not possible. For this purpose, one must rely on overt behavioral signs or tests of cognitive function in addition to the drug analysis.

Although a number of body tissues and fluids can be used for drug testing, the most common specimen is urine for the following reasons: (1) the collection of urine is not invasive, (2) large volumes can be collected easily, (3) drugs and their metabolites are generally present in higher concentrations in urine than in other tissues or fluids because of the concentrating function of kidneys, (4) urine is easier to analyze than blood and other tissues because of the usual absence of protein and cellular constituents, and (5) drugs and their metabolites are usually very stable in frozen urine, allowing long-term storage of positive samples.

There are also some disadvantages in using urine. Unless the specimen is collected under direct visual observation, there can be substitution of a "clean" urine sample for a "dirty" urine sample. Direct visual observation often is not pleasant for the person supplying the urine or the person watching. Many people find it difficult to urinate while being observed. Because of the social taboo of directly watching a person urinate, the observer often will not directly watch the collection of the urine, thereby permitting tampering with the sample. Ingenious techniques have been developed for substituting samples, including strapping a bag to the body containing a clean sample from which a catheter is run to the urethra so it appears that a sample is being collected directly from the patient. Samples also can be tampered with by dilution of the sample or by adding ions, such as salts, that may interfere with some testing procedures. Finally, if the collected urine is not carefully labeled and marked when it changes hands before the testing is done and there is not a clear chain of custody for the sample, the validity of the test can easily be challenged.

Urine drug testing should be carried out in a laboratory that is accredited by an appropriate accrediting agency, such as the Centers for Disease Control or the College of American Pathologists, and that engages in regular proficiency testing. The laboratory director should be a pathologist, other physician, toxicologist, or doctoral-level laboratory scientist who has extensive experience and background in analytic chemistry, clinical pharmacology, and/or forensic toxicology. The director should be qualified to interpret the results of the test procedures.

TESTING TECHNIQUES

Table 1 compares the various testing techniques that are used presently.[11] Techniques that require treatment of samples prior to analysis are more prone to technical error. When major instrumentation is needed, the expense of the procedure increases. As can be seen from Table 1, no single technique is totally satisfactory in meeting all needs.

One of the most common concerns about drug testing is the duration of detectability of drugs in urine following the last use of the drug, which depends on the methodologies employed and the drugs themselves. Table 2 shows the approximate duration of detectability of selected drugs in

Table 1.—Comparison of Commonly Used Analytic Techniques[††]

Technique*	Preanalysis Treatment of Sample	Major Instrumentation	Drug Identification	Can Specimen Be Adulterated	Limits of Sensitivity	Instrumentation Costs, $	Confirmation Required	Multiple Drug Analysis at Once	Level of Personal Experience
TLC	Yes	No	Position on plate	No	1 µg/mL	...	Yes	Yes	High
Modified TOXI-LAB	Yes	No	Response to color reagents fluorescent pattern	No	0.2-5 µg/mL	500	Yes	Yes	Moderate
HPLC with scanning ultraviolet detector	Yes	Yes	Relative retention times; comparison of ultraviolet spectra with standards	No	0.02-10 µg/mL	20 000-50 000	No†	Yes	High
Dual-column capillary GC with nitrogen detectors	Yes	Yes	Relative retention times matched in both columns; comparison of peaks with standards	No	0.01-10 µg/mL	20 000-50 000	No†	Yes	High
Capillary GC/MS	Yes	Yes	Relative retention times; comparison of mass spectra with standards	No	0.001-5 µg/mL	20 000-200 000	No	Yes	High
EMIT	No	Yes	Variation in enzyme activity	Yes	0.025-5 µg/mL	7000-100 000	Yes	No	Moderate
RIA	No	Yes	Variation of bound radiolabeled tracer	Yes	0.001-10 µg/mL	5000-100 000	Yes	No	Moderate
Color or spot tests	No	No	Response to color reagents	Yes	0.1-10 ng/nL	...	Yes	No	Moderate

*TLC indicates thin-layer chromatography; modified TOXI-LAB, modified thin-layer chromatography; HPLC, high-performance liquid chromatography; GC, gas chromatography; GC/MS, gas chromatography/mass spectrometry; EMIT, enzyme-multiplied immunoassay technique; and RIA, radioimmunoassay.
†Confirmation necessary only if results must meet a forensic challenge.

Table 2.—Approximate Duration of Detectability of Selected Drugs in Urine[12-27]

Drug	Approximate Duration of Detectability*	Limits of Sensitivity of Analytic Techniques (μmol/L)
Amphetamine	48 h	0.5 μg/mL (4)
Methamphetamine	48 h	0.5 μg/mL (3)
Barbiturates		
Short acting	24 h	
Hexobarbital		1.0 μg/mL (4)
Pentobarbital		0.5 μg/mL (2)
Secobarbital		0.5 μg/mL (2)
Thiamylal		1.0 μg/mL (4)
Intermediate acting	48-72 h	
Amobarbital		1.0 μg/mL (4)
Aprobarbital		1.5 μg/mL (7)
Butabarbital		0.5 μg/mL (2)
Butalbital		1.5 μg/mL (7)
Long acting	≥7 d	
Barbital		5.0 μg/mL (27)
Phenobarbital		1.0 μg/mL (4)
Benzodiazepines	3 d†	1.0 μg/mL (3)
Cocaine metabolites	2-3 d	
Benzoylecgonine		0.5 μg/mL (2)
Ecgonine methyl ester		1.0 μg/mL (3)
Methadone	≈3 d	0.5 μg/mL (1)
1,5-Dimethyl-3,3-diphenyl-2-ethylidene pyrrolidine (metabolite of methadone)		0.5 μg/mL (1)
Codeine	48 h	0.5 μg/mL (2)
Morphine		1.0 μg/mL (4)
Propoxyphene	6-48 h	0.5 μg/mL (1)
Norpropoxyphene		1.5 μg/mL (4)
Cannabinoids (11-nor-Δ9-tetra-hydrocannabinol-9-carboxylic acid)	3 d,‡ 5 d,§ 10 d,‖ 21-27 d¶	20 ng/mL (65)
Methaqualone	≥7 d	1.0 μg/mL (4)
Phencyclidine	≈8 d	0.5 μg/mL (2)

*Interpretation of the duration of detectability must take into account many variables, such as drug metabolism and half-life, subject's physical condition, fluid balance and state of hydration, and route and frequency of ingestion. These are general guidelines only.
†Using therapeutic dosages.
‡Single use.
§Moderate smoker (4 times/wk).
‖Heavy smoker (smoking daily).
¶Chronic heavy smoker.

urine and their limit of sensitivity for urine drug screening.[12-27]

Screening Techniques

Color or Spot Tests. One of the earliest tests for detecting drugs was the spot test, which is performed by adding a small amount of urine to a reagent that turns a specific color if the drug is present. This test is most useful for finding drugs that are not detected by some of the broad-spectrum techniques described later herein. The advantages of the spot test are that it is easy to perform, does not require elaborate technology, and can be applied directly to an aliquot of urine or other biologic fluid. It is inexpensive because most of the reagents are readily available. The results are immediate and the test can be read by the eye. By adding spectrophotometric equipment to the testing procedure, a semiquantitative analysis can be done.

The spot test has two important disadvantages, however. First, a large number of drugs or metabolites can cause similar color changes, making it difficult to identify the exact compound present. Second, a relatively high concentration of a drug is needed to form the color reactions with the reagent. These two problems result in relatively high rates of false-positive and false-negative results. This type of test is most applicable when testing for salicylates,[28] ethchlorvynol (Placidyl)[29] and ethyl alcohol.[30]

Thin-layer Chromatography. Thin-layer chromatography (TLC) was one of the first analytic techniques used to screen for a broad spectrum of drugs. A number of different procedures have been developed over the years, with increasing versatility, sensitivity, and ease of operation.[31-35] Because of these developments, TLC probably is the analytic technique most applicable for broad-spectrum drug screening.   One major drawback of TLC techniques is that they require extraction and concentration of the sample to enable the drugs and metabolites to be removed from the myriad of endogenous compounds that may interfere with the sample's migration and identification. There are other drawbacks as well. It is not easy to save the detection information on hard copy, because photographic representations of the plate at each stage of detection do not reproduce the colors very satisfactorily. Also, the drugs may stain somewhat differently, depending on how fresh the reagents are, and the spots must be interpreted quickly by the eye before colors fade and before further staining is done to identify other types of drugs. Although it is rare that the two drugs have the same migration or color characteristics, when this does occur it produces false-positive results. Finally, because of the broad range of drugs that TLC detects, it is not very specific, and other techniques must be used for confirmation.

Immunoassays. In the past few years, immunoassay techniques have been widely used to detect drugs. These techniques are based on the ability to produce antibodies to various drugs. The two most commonly employed techniques are the radioimmunoassay and the enzyme-multiplied immunoassay technique.

Radioimmunoassay is based on the principle that a drug labeled with a radioactive substance competes for the antibody binding site with the same drug not labeled with a radioactive substance. The more unlabeled drug there is in the sample, the less radioactive drug binds to the antibody. After all reagents are mixed, the drug-antibody complex is precipitated and the radioactivity is measured in the supernatant. Because the level of radioactivity can be measured, these tests are semiquantitative. Radioimmunoassay can be used to detect opiates, barbiturates, amphetamines, benzoylecgonine (a cocaine metabolite), phencyclidine, cannabinoids, and LSD.

There are several problems with radioimmunoassays: (1) special training in the use of radioactive substances is required, and the laboratory must have an expensive gamma counter to analyze the radioactivity; (2) these tests are discrete, that is, only one drug may be tested for at a time; (3) if the urine is tampered with by the addition of various adulterants, uniformly false-negative results may be produced; and (4) linearity of response and cross-reactivity with other drugs may produce both false-positive and false-negative results.[36]

The enzyme-multiplied immunoassay technique is used more commonly than the radioimmunoassay technique. Its advantages are that it is rapid and semiquantitative and it can detect a number of drugs, including opiates, barbiturates, amphetamines, cocaine and its metabolites, benzodiazepines, methaqualone, methadone, phencyclidine, and cannabinoids. Most of the instruments used in this technique are inexpensive.

The disadvantages of this technique are the expense of the reagents and the limited sources from which they are available. Urine specimens also can be adulterated to produce universally false-negative results. Other problems include difficulty with linearity of response and cross-reactivity with other drugs. It is not possible to predict which other drugs or metabolites may cross-react. For example, by chance the non-steroidal anti-inflammatory agents were found to cross-react with cannabinoids, amphetamines, and barbiturates. This technique was altered to eliminate these cross-reactivities. Table 3 shows possible cross-reactivity of tested drugs with commonly used prescription and nonprescription medications when radioimmunoassay and enzyme-multiplied immunoassay procedures are employed.[37]

Because of the limitations of both of these techniques, confirmatory tests are always required for positive results. Confirmation must not include another immunoassay technique.

A recent addition to the immunoassay procedures is fluorescence polarization immunoassay. Advantages of this technique are its ease of operation, its speed, and its ability to yield quantitative results automatically. Because the urinary concentrations of most drugs that are tested

Table 3.—Potential Cross-reactive Prescription and Nonprescription Medications in Radioimmunoassay or Enzyme-Multiplied Immunoassay Tests[37]

Test Substance	Possible Cross-reactors
Amphetamines	Diethylpropion
	Dopamine
	Ephedrine
	Fenfluramine
	p-Hydroxyamphetamine
	Isoxsuprine
	1-Methamphetamine
	Methylphenidate
	Nylidrin
	Phentermine
	Phenylephrine
	Phenylpropanolamine
	Propylhexedrine
	Pseudoephedrine
Barbiturates	Glutethimide
	Phenytoin
Opiates	Chlorpromazine
	Codeine
	Dextromethorphan
	Diphenoxylate
	Hydromorphone
	Meperidine
	Oxycodone
	d-Propoxyphene
Phencyclidine	Chlorpromazine
	Dextromethorphan
	Diphenhydramine
	Doxylamine
	Meperidine
	Thioridazine

are found in the mid-range of the operational capability of this procedure, rather than near its lower limit of detectability, this technique is also highly sensitive. However, it is susceptible to sample adulteration, it is expensive, and, at present, it is limited in availability.

New products have appeared that offer urine testing of drugs directly to the lay public. These kits claim to make use of enzyme immunoassay procedures, which are performed after a specimen is mailed to a laboratory. These tests are marketed as a means for parents to detect drug use in their children or for employees to determine if they are at risk for detection, among other purported uses.

The use of these tests is fraught with problems. In addition to cross-reactivity, false-positivity, and susceptibility to adulteration that are present in all immunoassays, there are problems of lack of chain of custody, long specimen-transit times in the mail, unknown temperature conditions while in transit, unknown quality control in the receiving laboratory, and possibly the lack of competent medical expertise for the interpretation of results. "Positive" results probably would not be followed up by any confirmatory testing. The scientific and clinical bases for the valid use of these tests are questionable.

Confirmation Techniques

Gas Chromatography. Gas chromatography is one of the most sensitive and specific techniques for detecting drugs in body fluids.[38-40] In recent years, new technology has allowed the use of dual, small-bore capillary columns in the gas chromatographic procedures, as well as new types of detectors, which increase the sensitivity and specificity of the procedure even more. The criterion used to establish identity of a compound using this technique is a matching of the retention time (i.e., time from injection of a substance into the chromatograph until the substance elutes) of the unknown compound with that of the pure, known substance within a window of 0.05 minutes for each column. With proper application, the rate of false-positive results is less than 0.01%.[41]

Despite the high specificity, there are several drawbacks associated with gas chromatography. The first is the expense of the equipment and the need for highly trained personnel. Second, only one sample can be run at a time, making it much slower than most of the other testing techniques. Because two different types of columns as well as long temperature programs (i.e., increasing the temperature to elute first the volatile and then the less volatile drugs) have to be used to identify many different drugs, this procedure is usually unsuitable for mass screening. However, gas chromatography has been used successfully to screen for hypnotics and sedatives,[42] nitrogen-containing drugs,[43] and volatile and nonvolatile alkaloids[44] in situations when sensitivity, specificity, and breadth of the procedure take precedence over speed. Gas chromatography is an excellent method for confirming the presence of drugs detected by more sensitive and broad screening procedures in a clinical, non-forensic setting.

Gas Chromatography/Mass Spectrometry. One of the most specific tools for testing drugs is the technique of combining gas chromatography with mass spectrometry.[39-40] Gas chromatography/mass spectrometry combines the chemical separating power of the gas chromatograph with the molecular identifying power of the mass spectrometer. In its scanning mode, the gas chromatograph separates the compounds of the biologic extract and the mass spectrometer breaks down the eluting compounds into electrically charged ion fragments. Different compounds break down into different fragment patterns and, like fingerprints, no two fragment patterns are alike. The computer system controlling gas chromatography/mass spectrometry can match the fragmentation pattern of unknowns with analytic standards. The mass spectrometer also has a selected ion-monitoring mode that markedly increases the sensitivity of detecting low concentrations of compounds and is the most commonly used method for forensic confirmation of both the presence and the amount of drugs and metabolites isolated from biologic specimens.

One of the major drawbacks to all gas chromatographic techniques is the time it takes to prepare the sample before testing. Unless this is done properly, the results can be highly inaccurate. Furthermore, the gas chromatography mass spectrometry equipment is enormously expensive, can process only one sample at a time, and requires a highly trained operator, thereby making this procedure beneficial only as a confirmatory procedure. Based on its accuracy, gas chromatography/mass spectrometry is the procedure that is most often used in forensic work.

High-Performance Liquid Chromatography. High-performance liquid chromatography has good sensitivity and high specificity. As with gas chromatography, an extraction of the drugs from the urine must be performed, and derivatives of the drug in question must be formulated with certain other substances to increase the sensitivity for detection. A recent improvement in the detection capabilities of high-performance liquid chromatography has markedly increased its discriminating power. Diode array/ultraviolet-visible spectral detectors permit capture of a complete ultraviolet-visible spectrum at several points on an eluting peak. Like a mass spectrometer in scanning mode, these ultraviolet-visible spectra can be matched by computer to the spectra of pure analytic standards, giving this procedure a high degree of specificity. Because of the expense of the equipment and the need for preparation, this technique is most applicable for confirming positive results from other screening techniques, although its acceptability in forensic settings has not been firmly established. Care must be taken to ensure that samples and controls are run under identical conditions. As the price of high-performance liquid chromatography equipment decreases, it will be used more widely.

CONCLUSIONS

Physicians should be familiar with the strengths and limitations of drug screening techniques and programs. Due to the limited specificity of the inexpensive and widely available screening techniques, forensically acceptable testing programs must include highly specific, technically more complicated, and more expensive confirmation techniques, which unequivocally establish the identities and quantities of drugs. Results from such drug testing programs can yield accurate evidence of prior exposure to drugs. Drug testing does not provide any information about patterns of drug use, about abuse of or dependence on drugs, or about mental or physical impairments that may result from drug use.

Physicians need to be aware of the objectives of a drug testing program in which they participate, and they should be satisfied that the selection of subjects to be tested and the screening and confirming techniques that are used meet the objectives. Since physicians often are called on to interpret results, they should be familiar with the pharmacokinetic properties of the drugs to be tested and the use to which the results will be put.

From the Council on Scientific Affairs, the American Medical Association, Chicago, IL.

Report J of the Council on Scientific Affairs, adopted by the House of Delegates of the American Medical Association, as amended in lieu of Resolutions 84 and 106, at the 1986 Interim Meeting.

This report is not intended to be construed or to serve as a standard of medical care. Standards of medical care are determined on the basis of all of the facts and circumstances involved in an individual case and are subject to change as scientific knowledge and technology advance and patterns of practice evolve. This report reflects the views of the scientific literature as of December 1986.

Reprint requests to Council on Scientific Affairs, American Medical Association, 535 N. Dearborn St., Chicago, IL 60610 (William R. Hendee, PhD)

REFERENCES

1. Chamberlain J: Analysis of Drugs in Biological Fluids. Boca Raton, FL, CRC Press Inc, 1985, pp 122-125.
2. Caplan YH: Analytical techniques, in Baselt RC(ed): Introduction to Forensic Toxicology. Davis, Calif, Biomedical Publications, 1981, pp 161-162.
3. Kogan JD: Expert testimony, in Baselt RC(ed): Introduction to Forensic Toxicology. Davis, CA, Biomedical Publications, 1981, pp 247-274.
4. Henion J, Covey T, Maylin G: Forensic mass spectrometry in equine drug testing. Spectra 1985; 10:21-28.
5. Dogoloff LI, Angarola RT, Price SC: Urine Testing in the Workplace. Rockville, MD, American Council for Drug Education, 1985.

6. Biasotti AA, Valentine TE: Blood alcohol concentration determined from urine samples as a practical equivalent or alternative to blood and breath alcohol tests. J Forensic Sci 1985;30:194-207.

7. Payne JP, Hill DW, King NW: Observations on the distribution of alcohol in blood, breath and urine. Br Med J 1966;1:196-202.

8. Morgan WHD: Concentrations of alcohol in samples of blood and urine taken at the same time. J Forensic Sci Soc 1965;5:15-21.

9. Heise HA: Concentrations of alcohol in samples of blood and urine taken at the same time. J Forensic Sci 1967;12:454-462.

10. Payne JP, Foster DV, Hill DW, et al: Observations on interpretation of blood alcohol levels derived from analysis of urine. Br Med J 1967;3:819-823.

11. Bittirofer JA, Benton B: Rapid Drug Screening in the Hospital Clinic Laboratory. Kansas City, MO, Marion Laboratories Inc, 1982.

12. Baselt RC: Disposition of Toxic Drugs and Chemicals in Man, ed 2. Davis, CA, Biomedical Publications, 1982.

13. Gorodetsky CW: Detection of drugs of abuse in biological fluids. Handbook Exp Pharmacol 1977; 45:319-409.

14. Clarke EG(ed): Isolation and Identification of Drugs. London, The Pharmaceutical Press, 1969, vol 1.

15. Rutter ER: Automated method for screening urine for amphetamine and some related primary amines. Clin Chem 1972;18:616-620.

16. Parker KD, Elliot HW, Wright JA, et al: Blood and urine concentrations of subjects receiving barbiturates, meprobamate, glutethimide, or diphenylhydantoin. Clin Toxicol 1970;3:131-145.

17. Ravn-Jonsen A, Luding M, Secher O: Excretion of phenobarbitone in urine after intake of large doses. Acta Pharmacol Toxicol 1969;27:193-201.

18. Waters N, Gaha TJ, Reynolds I: Random urine analysis from drug addicts in a methadone treatment programme.Med J Aust 1975;2:170-172.

19. Van Dyke C, Byck R, Barash PG, et al: Urinary excretion of immunologically reactive metabolite(s) after intranasal administration of cocaine, as followed by immunoassay. Clin Chem 1977;23:241-244.

20. Hamilton HE, Wallace JE, Shimek ELJr, et al: Cocaine and benzoylecgonine excretion in humans. J Forensic Sci Soc 1977;22:697-707.

21. Lui CT, Adler FL: Immunological studies on drug addiction: Antibodies reactive with methadone and their use for detection of the drug. J Immunol 1973;111:472-477.

22. Amundson ME, Johnson ML, Manthey JA: Urinary excretion of d-propoxyphene hydrochloride in man. J Pharm Sci 1965;54:684-686.
23. Levine S: EMIT dau and EMIT st Urine Cannabinoid Assays: Accuracy, Passive Inhalation and Detection Time in Clinical Studies. Palo Alto, CA, Syva Co, 1983.
24. Dackis CA, Pottash ALC, Annitto W, et al: Persistence of urinary marijuana levels after supervised abstinence. Am J Psychiatry 1982;139:1196-1198.
25. Kogan MJ, Jukofsky D, Verebey K, et al: Detection of methaqualone in human urine by radio immunoassay and gas-liquid chromatography after a therapeutic dose. Clin Chem 1978;24:1425-1426.
26. Gupta RC, Lu I, Oei GL, et al: Determination of phencyclidine (PCP) in urine and illicit street samples. Clin Toxicol 1975;8:611-621.
27. Ellis GM: Excretion patterns of cannabinoid metabolites after last use in a group of chronic users. Clin Pharmacol Ther 1985;38:572-578.
28. Trinder P: Rapid determination of salicylate in biological fluids. Biochem J 1954;57:301-303.
29. Frings CS, Cohen PS: Rapid colorimetric method for the quantitative determination of ethchlorvynol (Placidyl) in serum and urine. Am J Clin Pathol 1970;54:833-836.
30. Kozelka FL, Hine CH: Method for the determination of ethyl alcohol for medicolegal purposes. Ind Engl Analyt Chem Educ 1941;13:905.
31. Sunshine I: Use of thin-layer chromatography in the diagnosis of poisoning. Am J Clin Pathol 1963;40:576-582.
32. Sunshine I, Fike WW, Landesman H: Identification of therapeutically significant organic bases by thin-layer chromatography. J Forensic Sci 1966;11:428-439.
33. Davidow B, Li Petri N, Quame B: A thin-layer chromatographic screening procedure for detecting drug abuse. Am J Clin Pathol 1968;50:714-719.
34. Heaton AM, Blumberg AG: Thin-layer chromatographic detection of barbiturates, narcotics, and amphetamines in urine of patients receiving psychotropic drugs. J Chromatogr 1969;41:367-370.
35. Kaistha KK, Jaffe JH: TLC techniques for identification of narcotics, barbiturates, and CNS stimulants in a drug abuse urine screening program. J Pharm Sci 1972;61:679-689.
36. Chamberlain J: Analysis of Drugs in Biological Fluids. Boca Raton, Fla, CRC Press Inc, 1985, pp 115-136.

66 Use of the Laboratory

37. Baselt RC: Urine drug screening by immunoassay: Interpretation of results, in Baselt RC(ed): Advances in Analytical Toxicology. Foster City, CA, Biomedical Publications, 1984, vol 1, pp 81-123.
38. Mule SJ: Routine identification of drugs of abuse in human urine: I. Application of fluorometry, thin-layer and gas-liquid chromatography. J Chromatogr 1971; 55:255-265.
39. Costello CE, Hertz HS, Sakai T, et al: Routine use of a flexible gas chromatography-mass spectrometer-computer system to identify drugs and their metabolites in body fluids of overdose victims. Clin Chem 1974;20:255-265.
40. Ullucci PA, Cadoret R, Stasiowski PD, et al: A GC/MS drug screening procedure in current use. Clin Chem 1976;22:1197-1198.
41. Frethold D, Joves P, Sebrosky G, et al: Testing for basic drugs in biological fluids by solvent extraction and dual capillary GC/NPD. J Anal Toxicol 1986;10:10-14.
42. Newton B, Foery RF: Retention indices and dual capillary gas chromatography for rapid identification of sedative hypnotic drugs in emergency toxicology. J Anal Toxicol 1984;8:129-134.
43. Hime GW, Bednarczyk LR: Identification of basic drugs in urine by dual fused silica capillary column GC. J Anal Toxical 1982;6:247-249.
44. Kvoppasalmi K, Karjalainen V: Doping Analysis in Helsinki 1983: The First IAAF World Championships. Helsinki. Clinical Chemistry Research Foundation Library, 1984, vol 1.

Chapter 5

REFERRAL

The primary care physician entrusted with the day-to-day treatment of adolescents must accept a major responsibility for the diagnosis, treatment, and referral to specialty care of those patients whose medical difficulties are caused or complicated by drug involvement. Deciding when to refer these patients to specialized drug treatment programs, which programs are best, and how to prepare families and adolescents for successful transition into the specialty program are perplexing clinical issues.

The first challenge for the physician is to determine the severity of the adolescent's drug involvement. Many surveys have shown drug use to be quite common; thus, the degree of habituation, addiction, and destructiveness for each individual user requires careful evaluation. This evaluation is complicated by the fact that one symptom of serious drug involvement is denial. This denial is a genuine psychological phenomenon; it is not a simple conscious misrepresentation that stems from the adolescent's anxiety that he/she will get into trouble by confessing to drug use. The process of denial actually convinces the adolescent that his/her drug use is not a serious problem, even when objective observation would suggest very serious impairment. From a practical point of view, denial creates a situation in which one cannot depend on the personal report of the patient about his/her illness. It deprives the health-care professional of one of his/her most important sources of information. The denial process also frequently has an impact on the family, causing parents to underestimate their child's drug involvement to a significant degree. Moreover, it means that they too cannot be counted upon for information regarding the severity of their child's drug use. Despite these difficulties, the physician should not ignore input from the patient and the family or dismiss it out of hand. It is merely to suggest that some skepticism is wise and that an assessment of other related factors is also important. These factors include:

1. **Age at which the child began to use drugs.** Even adolescents who claim that they do not use drugs frequently may give accurate information regarding the age at which they first used them. Early onset of drug use suggests more serious involvement, since it is frequently correlated with a greater degree of personal or family disturbance. Early drug use also causes a longer disruption of normal psychological and educational development because of the effects of intoxication, withdrawal from parents and other adults, and interference with motivation.

2. **Assessment of the patient's peer group.** This assessment should focus not only on the nature of the emotional relationships between the patient and his/her friends but also on whether the friends are drug-involved. If the adolescent has maintained close relationships with nondrug-using friends, this is a more positive sign than if he/she has become completely immersed in a drug-oriented peer group. Evidence of a shift toward a more drug-oriented peer group in the adolescent also suggests a more serious problem. Information from both the patient and parents should be used in assessing the peer group.

3. **Assessment of the patient's relationship with his/her family.** Severe drug involvement usually leads to alienation and often to hostility and rebelliousness toward parental figures. The basic family strength and its capacity to be supportive and helpful in the treatment effort as well as the youngster's willingness to permit the family to be involved, will influence referral decisions.

4. **The adolescent's attitude toward drug use.** If the adolescent defends his/her drug involvement and has little interest in curtailing it, treatment will be much more difficult. On the other hand, if the adolescent

shows mixed feelings and questions the wisdom of drug use, this is a positive sign. It is not encouraging if the adolescent merely admits to excessive drug use and describes plans to reduce drug intake. Good intentions are common among substance abusers and they rarely result in lasting improvement.

5. **The presence or absence of other psychiatric, developmental, or educational problems.** In general, the more complex the clinical picture, the more likely the child is to require referral to a specialist.

6. **Quantity and type of drugs used and frequency of drug use.** To the extent it is available, this information is valuable in determining the severity of the problem and the likelihood that special treatment is necessary.

7. **The relative importance in the adolescent's life of chemical agents as opposed to relationships with people and human values.** This is the most important assessment consideration of all. The degree to which the adolescent is willing to sacrifice relationships with others and his/her own future in order to continue drug use is a crucial measure of the extent of habituation or addiction.

8. **The presence of organ dysfunction secondary to drug use.** Secondary symptoms suggest that the adolescent's capacity to consider his/her own well-being above his/her preoccupation with drug use has been seriously impaired.   Although these factors may sound somewhat complicated, they fall into rather clear patterns in the context of a review of the entire clinical situation.

OFFICE TREATMENT OF DRUG-INVOLVED ADOLESCENTS

Some adolescents whose problems are not severe may be managed by the primary care physician. Among these patients would be those whose drug involvement was of relatively late onset, those who maintain relationships with friends who do not use drugs, those with positive family bonds, and those with some desire to become drug-free. Even in the best of cases, successful treatment requires long-term involvement and follow-up by the primary care physician. Periodic appointments with the adolescent and with one or both parents to review the patient's progress and provide the necessary support and supervision are essential. Continued medical and educational input from the physician as well as his/her active interest in the patient's constructive social activities and support to the family can reinforce strengths within the patient and the family and thereby facilitate improvement. It is frequently wise to insist on periodic monitored drug urinalysis, since this can provide clear and unambivalent evidence of an abstinence from drug use. Obviously, if an adolescent still wishes to use drugs, he or she can do so and simply plan a period of abstinence in advance of the office visit. However, many adolescents utilize the drug test as a reinforcement for that side of their personality that desires to remain drug-free. In other words, the issue is not one of trusting or not trusting the adolescent but of attempting to join the adolescent in the battle against a very tricky and untrustworthy "enemy within"—the adolescent's habituation or addiction to drugs. It is also usually advisable to refer the patient and the family to local self-help groups, particularly if such groups are interested in and experienced with dealing with adolescents who have drug problems. Among the largest and most helpful are Alcoholics Anonymous and Narcotics Anonymous. These well-established self-help organizations have chapters in most locations in the country. The physician will need to inquire about their willingness to accept adolescent substance abusers.

PATIENTS WHO REQUIRE REFERRAL TO SPECIALTY TREATMENT

Patients who do not succeed in office treatment will obviously require referral. This possibility should be discussed at the outset of office management. The physician may say, "This is a potentially serious problem, and sometimes it cannot be overcome without very extensive treatment. However, some people have been able to successfully deal with the problem with my help. Let's try the simpler method first and evaluate its success." The office management should be deemed a failure if the patient continues to use drugs. This bold statement can be made safely, because if the drug use is not a genuine problem, it is very unlikely that the family or the physician will know that it continues. If it comes to light, one is probably only seeing the "tip of the iceberg." Some patients should be referred to specialty care immediately. These include adolescents with an early onset of drug use, a long history of heavy involvement, immersion in a drug-oriented peer group, and severe family disruptions. Those with accompanying emotional or psychiatric problems should likewise be referred immediately.

DISCOVERY AND EVALUATION OF SPECIALTY PROGRAMS

The primary care physician needs to become familiar with the drug-abuse treatment resources available in his/her community. Information can be solicited from the local medical society, Alcoholics Anonymous, Narcotics Anonymous, and national clearinghouses such as the National Clearinghouse for Alcohol and Drug Information (NCADI) at P.O. Box 2345, Rockville, MD 20852 (301-468-2600). These organizations may provide names of mental health practitioners who have special expertise in the treatment of drug-involved adolescents. Unfortunately, one cannot assume that all mental health practitioners have the requisite skills for managing adolescents who abuse drugs, even though they may be quite effective in treatment of young people with emotional problems uncomplicated by drug use. The referral process works best if the primary care physician has some direct knowledge of the specialty program and is able to recommend it with confidence and enthusiasm. Each program must be evaluated according to the knowledge and preference of the individual physician, but it may be useful to consider the following questions:

1. Does the program center around an expectation of total abstinence? Most experts in drug treatment agree that only programs requiring total abstinence have a proven success rate.

2. Does the program address the addictive process directly? Are there licensed drug counselors to supervise effective group confrontations and drug-education experiences in the program?

3. Does the program have a family component that acknowledges the importance of parent involvement in treatment?

4. Does the program make adequate provisions for the fact that serious drug involvement is a chronic illness? Short-term programs that promise too much should be regarded with some suspicion unless they are associated with follow-up programs that offer long-term support to the drug-free youth.

PREPARATION FOR REFERRAL

The parents are the critical element in successful referral. If the parents have become convinced that there is indeed a serious problem and can be assured that effective therapies exist, they are likely to take responsibility for ensuring that treatment actually occurs. Drug-using adolescents, particularly those with problems serious enough to require specialty treatment, often are not dependable allies in the referral process. Like the adult alcoholic, the seriously drug-involved adolescent usually goes for treatment only because of external pressure and under some duress. At times, the severity of the adolescent's resistance can be diminished through a process of gentle confrontation with the reality of the severity of the problem, a technique that is often referred to as an "intervention." However, the adolescent's denial, rationalization, and minimalization of the problem will frequently erode any desire for treatment that might be elicited through such an approach. The adolescent should be told directly that he/she requires treatment and that it is being recommended. It is sometimes necessary to be less than specific if an adolescent's immediate safety is at risk or if an attempt to commit suicide or to run away or another life-threatening event might follow the discussion of treatment. Again, the parents must take major responsibility for arranging the adolescent's entry into treatment.

TYPES OF THERAPY

Conventional psychotherapy is often ineffective in the treatment of severely drug-involved adolescents. Psychotherapy requires a capacity to invest emotionally in the therapist and to report honestly actions and feelings that are creating problems. The drug-involved adolescent finds this honesty and trust very difficult to establish. The concept that adolescents use drugs because they are emotionally disturbed and that removal of the underlying emotional problems by psychotherapy will cure them ignores the complexity of habituation and addiction. In other words, even if the problem began as an emotional problem, it is now a toxicological, pharmacological, biochemical, sociological, and spiritual problem that will not usually yield to psychotherapy alone. On the other hand, psychotherapy as an adjunct to other drug-treatment approaches, particularly if administered by a therapist who is familiar with the realities of drug involvement, can be extremely valuable. There are several types of treatment programs specifically designed for drug involvement. Outpatient drug programs often combine family therapy, education about the psychological and physical effects of heavy drug use, and group therapy focused on the drug problem. These programs are beneficial if the drug use is only moderate and if the family is dependable and cooperative.

Severe drug use usually requires a period of external supervision that can be arranged through hospitalization, placement in a residential drug treatment center, or a special program that uses family members and former drug users to supervise the adolescent after use of drugs has been curtailed.

HOSPITAL TREATMENT

Psychiatric hospitalization can be useful in some cases in order to detoxify the patient and to begin the treatment and rehabilitation process. Hospital programs are much more effective if they meet the treatment criteria described above. Planning for appropriate aftercare is especially important. Hospitalization is usually indicated when the problem is severe, the adolescent is poorly motivated, the family needs extensive preparation, and, especially, if the young person has psychiatric problems that complicate the drug problem. Some inpatient programs are prepared to accept and treat even strongly resistant adolescents. Even though this group is difficult to treat, their illness is so malignant that even heroic efforts are worth trying. Approximately 50% of such patients do respond to treatment.

Residential treatment centers (RTCs) provide for longer term treatment of the drug-involved adolescent. Usually RTCs are not based on a medical model but are therapeutic communities often staffed by graduates of that program. The patients themselves take major responsibility for running the treatment center, and admission requires a fairly high level of motivation on the part of the adolescent. RTCs are often used as the long-term aftercare component of hospital treatment once the family and the adolescent have reached the point where they can take greater responsibility for their own care. A list of residential drug treatment centers is available through the National Institute on Drug Abuse. Many communities do not have a treatment center; in this case, problems in family involvement in the treatment process related to geographic distance may have to be evaluated. A number of special programs for the treatment of drug-involved adolescents have evolved in response to the tremendous increase in referrals in the last two decades. Representative and perhaps best known of these somewhat controversial programs is Straight, Inc. These community-based programs use a combination of close supervision, drug education, and an active effort to alter value systems in order to rehabilitate these youngsters. They depend on large group activities (100 to 200 youngsters) to mobilize peer pressure in a positive direction and to create enthusiasm for a constructive lifestyle and repudiation of the so-called "drug, sex, and rock-n-roll" orientation to life.   It is particularly important that the primary care physician understand these treatment groups and their philosophies so that they can be accurately described to families and so that the reasons behind their techniques can be explained. Without proper preparation, some parents respond to these programs with strong negative feelings and anxiety. They may view them as "cult-like," too controlling, or "puritanical." The accusation is often made that these programs "brainwash" the adolescent. However, these programs have successfully treated hundreds of youngsters, and as mentioned above, they may be particularly effective for a specific subpopulation of adolescents who do not respond well to traditional treatment. It is well worth the practitioner's time to become familiar with these programs and to explore their potential contribution to his/her patients. The funding of drug treatment is very complicated, and parents often need advice as they make arrangements for appropriate care. Alcoholics Anonymous and Narcotics Anonymous are free of cost. Hospital treatment programs are frequently eligible for private insurance coverage. In the public sector, some state and local public hospitals have developed sound drug-treatment programs. Other agencies, such as the Department of Juvenile Services or educational centers, may fund treatment; however, to secure funding it is usually necessary for the parents to become advocates for their child and to pursue actively all of these possibilities. Family support groups such as Families Anonymous, Tough Love, and Al-Anon have among their members individuals who have discovered ways to obtain financial support for treatment.   Costs of treatment vary greatly. Hospital care, as a rule, is the most expensive on a short-term basis. Although the rate per day in hospitals tends to be high, the overall cost may not be great since the hospital stay may be short and the follow-up treatment may be relatively inexpensive. On the other hand, residential treatment programs tend to have a relatively low cost per day but are often designed to provide treatment over a two- or three-year period, making the total cost relatively high.

SUMMARY

The primary care physician can be of tremendous assistance to families in detecting, evaluating, and treating the drug-involved adolescent. This effectiveness can be expanded if primary care physicians take the time to familiarize themselves with local treatment programs and make themselves available to the family as knowledgeable and decisive agents in supporting the painful process of treatment for serious drug involvement.

Chapter 6

PREVENTION PROGRAMS

Over the past two decades, there have evolved a wide variety of programs—local, state, and national—aimed at preventing alcohol and drug use and abuse among young people. These programs range from national media campaigns to school curricula to pamphlets distributed in waiting rooms.* Because drug- and alcohol-abuse prevention programs are so pervasive, most patients and their parents will have been exposed to at least one of them, and a portion of what the patient and family know and believe about alcohol and drugs will have been derived from them.

There are three major reasons why the practitioner should be familiar with the rationale, objectives, and activities of these programs. First, as already suggested, familiarity with these programs provides insight into where the patient or his/her parents may be "coming from" in terms of their knowledge, attitudes, and beliefs about drugs and alcohol. Second, knowledge of program content provides the opportunity for the practitioner to reinforce the positive messages that many programs communicate or, conversely, to balance the effects of programs that may be providing erroneous or counterproductive information. Finally, as a community expert in health issues, the practitioner may be called upon to comment on the desirability of launching a given program. In such cases, a working knowledge of the issues involved is key to providing useful advice to parents, educators, government officials, and others.

---

*Defining precisely what is meant by a "program" is a continuing problem for drug- and alcohol-abuse theorists. For example, potentially powerful preventive measures such as warning labels on cigarette packages or restrictions on alcohol sales do not fit conventional notions of a "program." For the purposes of this chapter, a prevention "program" will be defined as any purposive activity or set of activities aimed at reducing the onset or maintenance of drug or alcohol use or abuse or at reducing the negative consequences of such behavior.

This chapter provides a broad review of the state-of-the-art in drug- and alcohol-prevention programming. First, a brief historical overview of the last two decades of prevention programming is presented. Next, current programs are reviewed in terms of their rationale, goals and objectives, and activities. Finally, a separate section is devoted to programs that seek to prevent drinking and driving, since such programs raise special issues.

It is important to note that this chapter will not answer the question "What works in prevention?" The answer to this question is still unclear, partly because of the relative newness of prevention as a programmatic technology and partly because of the failure of well-controlled scientific studies to provide evidence of the effectiveness of specific prevention strategies that have been studied to date.

HISTORICAL OVERVIEW

In order to understand the diversity of current approaches to drug- and alcohol-abuse prevention, it is useful to briefly examine how prevention programs evolved. The modern history of prevention programs begins with initial responses to the "drug epidemic" of the late 1960s. The spread of "psychedelic" drug use, and to a lesser degree, amphetamine and barbiturate use, first on college campuses and later in the youth culture more generally, led to often hastily conceived attempts to reduce the numbers of youth who were "turning on, tuning in, and dropping out."

The earliest prevention programs of this period relied on moralizing, presentation of overblown and inaccurate information concerning the risks of drug use (so-called "scare tactic" programs), or both. Such approaches did little except impair credibility in the eyes of youth, who often knew (or thought they knew) more about drugs and their effects than the adult presenters. A more enlightened early approach was to present balanced, factual drug information (pharmacological, physical, psychological, and social effects; criminal justice issues) in an attempt to encourage rational decisions concerning drug use. Although such programs were more credible to youth than those based on scare tactics, subsequent research suggested that drug information alone did little to discourage use and that it may actually have been counterproductive. In particular, some data suggested that these programs served to arouse curiosity, to instruct youth in the finer points of drug use, or both, thus encouraging rather than discouraging drug experimentation.

As data on the correlates of drug use became available in the early 1970s, programs began to focus on the psychological traits and "life skills" that appeared to distinguish users from nonusers. These data suggested a relationship between drug use and variables such as low self-esteem, poor decision-making skills, and poor communication skills. It was not clear that low self-esteem, poor decision-making skills, or poor communication skills caused drug use; however, the reverse might have been true. Such correlate research, together with the then pervasive influence of the human potential movement in psychology, spawned the first "new generation" of preventive interventions—the affective education programs. These programs sought to improve self-esteem and decision-making and communication skills, and somewhat later, to aid youth in clarifying values regarding drug and alcohol use. Although the effectiveness of these programs has never been adequately demonstrated, some aspects of affective education remain a component of many drug and alcohol programs, particularly school-based programs.

More or less coincident with the emergence of the affective education programs, some drug-abuse theorists began to argue that the most effective way of preventing drug use was to provide access to "alternative highs" that would meet the same needs users claimed drugs met ("mind expansion," personal growth, excitement, challenge, relief from boredom) in nonpharmacological ways. Accordingly, programs were developed that provided youth with a variety of alternatives to drug use, ranging from wilderness challenges to community service to drug-free rock concerts. The alternative high terminology is no longer current, but the alternatives concept is still used in many prevention programs as a means for providing youth with enjoyable and safe recreation that is drug- and alcohol-free. One programmatic idea that derived from the alternatives movement—training youth to present prevention programs or provide counseling to other youth—is a component of some recent prevention initiatives.

Through much of the 1970s, the three program types just described—drug information, affective education, and alternatives—were dominant in prevention programming, and they remain so in many school-based prevention programs today. In the late 1970s, however, four new trends emerged that began to reshape drug and alcohol prevention. First, and perhaps most important, parents and communities nationwide began to mobilize grassroots prevention efforts that challenged the basic assumptions of existing programs. Leaders of these grassroots efforts believed that existing prevention programs were largely ineffective and that parents and concerned community leaders were in the best position to place controls on the drug-use behavior of youth. The activities of these individuals spawned two major programmatic initiatives— the concerned parents movement and the community prevention movement—that remain dominant forces in prevention.

In part as a result of the activities of concerned parents, a second major trend emerged—the doctrine of "responsible use." This doctrine, which was popular in the 1970s, held that certain substances, marijuana in particular, were not harmful to youth as long as they were used in ways that did not interfere with social or emotional functioning. Thus, the goal of prevention was to encourage youth to make responsible decisions with regard to substance use. Representatives of the concerned parents movement, along with some members of the scientific community, strongly questioned this doctrine on the grounds that any substance use posed unnecessary risks to developing youth, and by the 1980s, the doctrine of responsible use had largely disappeared from the prevention literature. Its disappearance brought with it the partial demise of many of the program approaches that had been pervasive in the 1970s, particularly those that sought to teach youth to make "responsible" decisions concerning substance use or that encouraged the development of "responsible" values. The third new trend in prevention arose from the growing recognition of the role that the peer group plays in the etiology of drug and alcohol abuse. The repeated research finding that substance-using youth have substance-using friends led to a plethora of programs based on the notion of "peer pressure" resistance. These programs ranged from relatively simplistic attempts to teach children to say "no" to drugs, to more complex interventions based in social-psychological theories of communication and persuasion. Extensive evaluation research must be undertaken to assess the effectiveness of these programs, for the research results concerning these programs has been mixed. There has been little convincing evidence that peer pressure is effective in preventing the onset of drug and alcohol use, although positive results in the prevention of cigarette smoking are regularly reported. It is important to note that these findings do not necessarily refute the etiologic role of peer influence. They do suggest the need for new theories concerning the mechanisms by which the peer group influences drug- and alcohol-related behavior that go beyond current notions of peer pressure.

The fourth new trend centers on the concept that prevention programs are most likely to be effective when they address multiple levels of influence. Many current theorists argue that factors that encourage drug and alcohol use are to be found at all levels of society, ranging from the advertising of the mass media to the influence of family and friends. Thus, it is argued, prevention programs that address a single level of influence will be undermined by influences from other levels and will necessarily be of limited effectiveness. Conversely, effective prevention programs will be those that are comprehensive and that involve interventions that address all levels of societal influence. Unfortunately, few examples of such programs have been implemented, partly because of the large commitment of resources required. Such programs are also among the most expensive to evaluate, and their effectiveness has yet to be scientifically assessed. Several research investigations are, however, currently under way that are examining the effectiveness of more than one prevention strategy implemented simultaneously. Results of such studies will provide at least a partial test of the validity of the multicomponent model. In summary, the history of drug- and alcohol-prevention programming has been one of shifting emphasis and emerging trends rather than dramatic breakthroughs. Today's programs represent amalgams of their predecessors, and with few exceptions (e.g., the doctrine of responsible use) programmatic ideas have been transformed rather than abandoned. The result has been a diverse tapestry of programmatic approaches with no single approach emerging as a dominant force.

REVIEW OF CURRENT PREVENTION PROGRAMMING

Current prevention theory recognizes that the risk factors that predispose to, reinforce, and enable drug and alcohol use and abuse are found at all levels of society. They are found within the biological and psychological makeup of the individual user, within the immediate environments of the family and the peer group, within the school and community, and within the larger social environment. In general, prevention programs focus largely on a single level of risk factors (e.g., the individual or the school) and their objectives and activities are designed to alter one or more factors within that level. Accordingly, one useful way to categorize prevention programs is in terms of the underlying program rationale (i.e., in terms of the risk factors addressed).*

Programs Focused On The Individual

Programs that focus on the individual generally view drug and alcohol use and abuse as arising as a result of one or more of six general classes of risk factors: 1) biological vulnerabilities; 2) need for affective regulation; 3) knowledge deficits; 4) skills deficits; 5) perceptions of invulnerability; and 6) sensation-seeking tendencies. As a group, prevention programs focused on individual risk factors are far and away the most common.

Biological Vulnerabilities

Programs based on theories of <u>biological vulnerabilities</u> are currently quite rare because of their relatively recent emergence as an area of interest in substance-abuse research. However, some investigators believe that ongoing research will suggest biological markers (genetic, biochemical, neurophysiological, or other) that can be used to identify individuals at risk of substance abuse or addiction.** If these investigators are correct, the numbers of such programs will likely increase in the future. The development of programs based on the detection of biologi-

---

*Some program rationales may not be supported by current theory (see chapter 1). However, supported or not, these rationales form the basis for program action.

**Despite considerable publicity in both the popular and scientific press, the findings of most studies suggesting biological markers for substance abuse are debatable. At this writing, the future utility of such research in developing prevention technologies cannot be accurately predicted.

cal markers poses a number of challenges for the prevention field. These include the problems associated with screening for any rare characteristic and the major problems associated with possible early labeling of children as "drug- or alcohol-problem-prone." Such programs present particular problems for prevention in the area of illicit drugs, since it is difficult to imagine a message that would be given to an "addiction-prone" youth (i.e., "Avoid all illicit drug use") that would not also be appropriate for youth in general.

It is likely that much of the burden of early detection based on biological markers (assuming useful markers are discovered) will rest with medical practitioners. The medical profession must therefore begin to consider the potential practice and ethical implications of this technology.

Affective Regulation

Related to programs based on biological vulnerabilities are those based on affective regulation theories. These posit that individuals use drugs and alcohol to self-medicate a variety of affective problems including depression, anxiety, boredom, and loneliness, or, similarly, that drug and alcohol abuse are secondary symptoms of primary personality disorders. Affective regulation programs rely on identifying individuals at risk and providing treatment or supportive counseling for the underlying problem. These programs pose some of the same problems discussed for biological vulnerability-based programs (e.g., problems associated with screening and the potential for labeling).

Knowledge Deficits

As suggested in the historical overview of prevention programming, programs based upon theories of knowledge deficit were among the earliest prevention efforts. These programs assume that individuals use or abuse drugs or alcohol because they lack accurate information concerning the detrimental effects of these substances. As suggested previously, there is little evidence to suggest that knowledge alone causes behavior change.* On the other hand, theorists generally agree that drug and alcohol knowledge is a useful precondition for behavior change, and thus many programs include basic information about the effects of drugs and alcohol. Programs aimed at overcoming knowledge deficits may be simple, one-shot efforts such as pamphlets or films, or they may be one segment of larger, more complex efforts such as school drug and alcohol curricula. Practitioners may wish to familiarize themselves with the materials being used in local programs in order to assess how these materials may have an impact on what patients and their parents "know" about drugs and alcohol.

Life Skills Deficits

Despite a general lack of evidence of the effectiveness of programs that seek to remediate life skills deficits (low self-esteem and poor decision-making and communication skills), such programs are still quite common. Indeed, the notion that low self-esteem and poor decision-making and communication skills are major precursors to drug and alcohol abuse is axiomatic among many prevention program planners. Accordingly, programs abound that are devoted to producing individuals with high self-esteem who are good communicators and good decision-makers. Remediation of life skills deficits is most commonly attempted in conjunction with remediation of knowledge deficits.

---

*A possible exception is in the area of cigarette smoking. In some studies, the reason children report for not smoking is fear of health consequences. However, as discussed later, it is impossible to positively link reductions in smoking with any single preventive intervention.

Invulnerability

Programs based on invulnerability theories proceed from the assumption that although young people may recognize the risks of drugs and alcohol, they do not believe that these risks are applicable to them ("It can never happen to me"). These programs attempt to motivate youth to avoid drugs and alcohol through fear arousal. Although the "scare tactic" programs of the early 1960s have given this technique a bad name, there is evidence that fear arousal that is based in scientific and legal facts and that is appropriate to the target audience can indeed have a positive impact on health-risk behavior. Some programs have attempted to overcome feelings of invulnerability by focusing on short-term risks that are salient to young people rather than on long-term risks that may be viewed as irrelevant. For example, smoking-prevention programs may focus on the way smokers smell (a social risk) rather than on the risk of cardiovascular disease, while drinking/driving prevention programs may focus on loss of driving privileges or the hassle and embarrassment of arrest rather than on accident statistics. Examples of programs focusing on immediate effects are the "counter-advertising" campaigns sponsored by Doctors Ought to Care (DOC) and the motivational materials used by Students Against Driving Drunk (SADD) and the multimedia drinking/driving presentation, Friday Night Live.

Sensation Seeking

The alternatives programs described in the historical overview (programs that sought to produce alternative highs) are examples of programs based on theories of sensation seeking—the theory that many people, especially youth, have a natural tendency to seek new, exciting, and sometimes risky experiences. Once fairly common, the numbers of programs that seek to provide alternative highs have diminished, although survival training and wilderness programs such as Outward Bound and Breakthrough Foundation are still in operation in some areas of the country. As discussed below, other types of alternatives programs are still quite common; however, both the theoretical rationale for and activities of such programs have changed.

Programs Focused On The Family

Prevention programs focused on the family view drug and alcohol use and abuse in terms of one or more of the following classes of risk factors: 1) family dynamics; 2) socialization or "habilitation" deficits; 3) negative parental modeling; and 4) lack of social control. These programs can be subdivided into those that are concerned largely with parent education and those that are concerned with the family as a whole. In practice, however, this distinction is often blurred.

Family Dynamics

Programs based on family dynamics theories appeal to a large body of correlate literature that associates increased risk of alcohol and drug abuse with such factors as parental permissiveness or inconsistency, loose family structure, harsh physical punishment, and poor family communication patterns. Accordingly, these programs seek to improve parenting skills and thus to indirectly reduce substance-abuse risk among children. A relevant and well-known example is Parent Effectiveness Training, which, although not designed as a drug- and alcohol-prevention program, has been adopted and adapted by the prevention field. Unfortunately, many parent-education programs have had difficulty recruiting participants, and it has been suggested that the parents who volunteer for such programs may not be those who need the program most.

Socialization Deficits

Related to programs based on family dynamics are those based on preventing or remediating socialization or habilitation deficits. These programs are based on the notion that the family is the major socialization agent, especially for young children, and that many modern families are failing to inculcate such basic values as self-control, self-motivation, and self-discipline. Accordingly, curricula for parents have been developed under the general rubric "Strengthening the Family" (after H. Stephen Glenn's book of the same name) that teach parents ways of structuring the home environment to increase the likelihood that children will develop these qualities.

Negative Parental Modeling

A third type of parent-education program are those that attempt to remediate negative parental modeling. These programs appeal to concepts from social learning theory that suggest that children's early notions concerning drugs and alcohol are learned by observing parents' behavior regarding alcohol, tobacco, over-the-counter and prescription medications, and, increasingly, marijuana and cocaine. The goal of these programs is to make parents aware of the impact of their substance-related behavior on their children and thus, to change parental behavior as a method for reducing youthful drug and alcohol risk. Programmatic interventions based on modeling are generally part of a larger parent-education program and are rarely seen alone except as public service announcements.

Social Control

Programs based on social control emerged as one component of the activities of concerned parents described in the historical overview. These programs proceed from the assumption that many parents have abdicated their responsibilities with regard to their children's drug and alcohol behavior. They seek to empower parents to reinstate social controls that will prevent or forestall experimentation with drugs and alcohol. The original core concept of such programs was the parent-peer support group, in which parents of children who associate with one another meet regularly to institute and enforce a consistent set of rules concerning curfews, parties, and other activities. Although some programs have experienced difficulties in maintaining parental interest in the parent-peer support group per se, these groups have often grown into broad-based, community prevention programs (see Chapter 2).

Programs Focused On The Peer Group

As suggested in the historical overview, the emergence of peer influence as a key risk factor in drug and alcohol abuse caused a major shift in the emphasis of many prevention programs. In general, programs focused on the peer group view peer influence as operating through one or more of three major mechanisms: 1) conformity to peer norms; 2) negative peer modeling; and 3) direct peer influence.

Conformity to Peer Norms

Programs based on conformity to peer norms derive from the assumption that a desire to "fit in the with crowd" is a major concern for adolescents. Thus, to the extent that using alcohol or drugs is considered normative ("in"), the general risk of such behavior is increased. Many programs have attempted to alter peer norms through strategies such as publicity campaigns that attempt to inculcate positive health messages into the youth culture or through "pledges" to remain drug- and alcohol-free (e.g., the current "Just Say No" campaign). Most surveys suggest that children believe that substance use is more common among their peers than it actually is. Accordingly, a limited number of programs (e.g., "Project Model Health" of the Wisconsin Division of Health) have attempted to give students information in actual local incidence and prevalence rates in order to foster the more realistic perception that substance abuse is not normative.

Negative Peer Modeling

Like programs based on parental modeling, programs derived from negative peer modeling theories proceed from the assumption that substance use and abuse are learned through modeling the behavior of salient others. These programs attempt to counteract or dilute negative peer models by exposing youth to attractive, positive models who communicate in words and actions an anti-substance use/abuse message. The programs employ youth or young adults, either live or on film, who model desired behaviors. Currently popular examples include "Project Smart" of the University of Southern California and the Children's Health Education Program of Tampa, Florida. Although these programs are enjoying wide popularity, their efficacy has not been proved.

Direct Peer Influence

Closely related to programs based on negative peer modeling theories are programs based on theories of direct peer influence. These programs proceed from the assumption that youth use drugs and alcohol because they are directly pressured to do so by peers. Accordingly, the programs teach "peer pressure resistance skills" that may range from simply saying "no" to drugs and alcohol to more complex, theory-based interventions. The "Just Say No" program is a recent example of the more simplistic programs; "Project Smart" an example of the more complex. As is the case with peer modeling programs, extensive evaluation research has failed to demonstrate the efficacy of such programs. Like the peer modeling programs, they nonetheless remain very popular.

Programs Focused On The School And Community

Unlike the programs discussed thus far, which tend to rely on psychological theory, programs focused on school and community risk factors appeal largely to sociological or ecological models of substance use and abuse. That is, they tend to locate the causes of substance abuse within the organizational characteristics of large social institutions* (e.g., the schools, the law enforcement system, the alcohol beverage control system). These programs generally address one or more of the following four risk factors: 1) inadequate deterrence; 2) availability; 3) negative social climate; and 4) poor social bonding.

Deterrence

Deterrence-based programs are probably among society's most ancient preventive responses to substance-use problems, with severe penalties for the use of certain substances (e.g., tobacco) recorded as early as the seventeenth century. In the 1970s, deterrence as a method for preventing substance use and abuse fell into disrepute, as many states liberalized their drug laws and many localities de-emphasized drug enforcement. Recently, however, there has been a resurgence of interest in deterrence-based programs. Of particular interest in the current con-

---

*A distinction should be made between programs that address risk factors located in the school and community and school- and community-based programs. The latter may address risk factors at any level, as when a school-based program provides drug information (individual level) or peer pressure resistance skills (peer level). The former address risk factors found specifically in the institution itself.

text is an emphasis on the importance of consistently enforced school drug and alcohol policies that stipulate a "no drug, no alcohol" campus policy, that articulate penalties for infractions, and that provide for equitable treatment of substance-involved youth. In general, research on deterrence-based programs suggests that such programs can have a dramatic but short-lived effect on use rates. Anecdotal evidence of the positive effects of school policies abounds; however, such results have not been researched systematically and the long-term effects of such policies are not known.

Availability

Many community-based programs have attempted to reduce the availability of substances to youth. These programs proceed from the assumption that reduced availability will lead to reduced consumption. The uniform 21-year-old alcohol purchase age legislation enacted at the national level represents one application of an availability model; local ordinances banning "head shops" are another. Currently, many communities are attempting to reduce alcohol availability to youth through controlling the numbers and types of retail outlets where alcohol may be purchased, educating and monitoring retail clerks and retail outlet owners, training servers in bars and restaurants and, most recently, cracking down on the availability of bogus identification cards. Although the effects of such programs are difficult to evaluate, existing data suggest that reduced availability does indeed reduce consumption and related problems.

Social Climate

Programs based on social climate are perhaps the broadest and most diffuse of prevention efforts. Indeed, rather than being classified as "programs," social climate manipulations are probably best conceptualized as the result of a number of programs acting in aggregate to promote a community-wide message. For example, increased law enforcement efforts, a strong school policy, the existence of a concerned parents group and "Just Say No" clubs, antidrug editorials in local newspapers, and the institution of drug education in the schools might, together, constitute a manipulation of a community's social climate with regard to drug and alcohol use and abuse. Community organization programs that attempt to involve as many community actors as possible in prevention (e.g., parents, youth, physicians, school personnel officers, police, local government officials, local media representatives) are the most common example of programs based on a social climate model. Social climate programs are extremely difficult to evaluate, and there is little evidence to support or refute their efficacy. Many theorists have appealed to social climate models to explain the decline in adult smoking, an effect that cannot be attributed to any single programmatic intervention.

Social Bonding

Originally developed by juvenile delinquency theorists, social bonding models maintain that antisocial behavior (including substance abuse) derives from a failure of some youth to "bond" to social institutions and their norms. This failure is largely ascribed to a failure of these youth to find (or be provided with) valued roles within the institutions. These youth have "nothing to lose" and hence, no reason to conform to normative proscriptions of antisocial acts.* Accordingly, substance-abuse prevention programs based

---

*Social bonding theorists have criticized the adoption of "no pass/no play" rules in school athletics on the grounds that youth who cannot achieve success in one arena (academics) are then prevented from achieving success in another arena (athletics), thus further reducing the probability that positive social bonding will occur.

on social bonding theories attempt to provide youth with opportunities to make a positive contribution to the community and to develop positive social bonds as a result. The earliest of such programs was "Channel One." Jointly sponsored by the National Institute on Drug Abuse and the Prudential Life Insurance Company, it provided youth with an opportunity to become involved in community service projects such as historical restorations, food cooperatives for the elderly, and youth job services. More recently, a variety of alternative activity programs have been developed that may be seen as outgrowths of the social bonding model. As suggested earlier, such programs have largely eclipsed alternatives programs based on alternative highs. Research on such programs in the substance-abuse area is sparse, but evidence from the juvenile delinquency prevention literature suggests that social bonding is a potentially powerful prevention strategy.

Programs Focused On The Larger Social Environment

Like programs based on school and community risk factors, programs that address drug and alcohol risk factors in the larger social environment generally appeal to sociological and/or ecological explanations of substance-related behavior. Indeed, many of the program models described under school and community programs (i.e., deterrence, availability, social climate) have been applied to the larger social environment, with the major difference being one of institutional focus (e.g., federal laws as opposed to local ordinances). One class of risk factors, however, clearly belongs to the larger social environment—those associated with mass media.* These include

---

*Again, a distinction must be made between programs that use the mass media as a programmatic tool and programs that address risk factors found in the media themselves. As is the case for school and community programs, the mass media may be a **vehicle** for prevention programming aimed at any level of risk factor. Indeed, most mas media campaigns are designed to affect the individual, the family, or the peer group.

risk factors associated with: 1) advertising of psychoactive substances; and 2) portrayal of substance use.

Advertising

The role of advertising in promoting drug and alcohol use and abuse is debatable, and few research studies exist to support either side of the debate. However, there are good theoretical reasons to expect that advertising might promote use, and three types of programs have been developed to counteract such potential negative effects. First, attempts have been made to limit, reduce, or eliminate cigarette and alcohol advertising.* Second, attempts have been made to develop "counter-advertising." Counter-advertisements such as those developed by Doctors Ought to Care (DOC) lampoon both the format and content of popular advertisements (e.g., an attractive model with a cigarette in his nose who claims, "I smoke for smell") or other promotional activities (e.g., an "Emphysema Slims" tennis tournament). Finally, some programs have attempted to educate youth about advertising techniques, to aid them in critiquing the persuasive messages in advertisements, or both. An example of this strategy is the "Life Skills Training" program, which devotes two sessions to media influences and advertising techniques. To date, there has been little research on either counter-advertising or advertising education to allow an assessment of their potential as prevention strategies. The pervasiveness of advertising in our society suggests that further exploration is justified.

Portrayal of Substance Use

Recently, there has been both scientific and popular concern over the portrayal of substance use in mass media.

---

*This strategy is an excellent example of a program that does not fit with traditional definitions of "program."

These concerns derive in part from the sheer numbers of hours youth devote to watching and listening to mass media (particularly television) and in part from the social modeling concerns discussed earlier in terms of family and peers. For example, content analyses of prime-time television programs have suggested that the portrayal of alcohol use does not generally provide a balanced view of the positive and negative aspects of drinking. This observation has led some researchers to attempt to educate television writers, producers, and directors about the alcohol messages their productions convey and to attempt to aid these individuals in presenting a more realistic picture of drinking. This approach is exemplified by the "Cooperative Consultation" process pioneered by Warren Breed and James DeFoe. Similarly, some individuals have become concerned about possible prodrug messages in popular music, although the scientific basis for such concerns is murky at best. These individuals have supported legislation that would require labeling of records to allow parents some control over the messages to which their children are allegedly exposed.

Drinking/Driving Prevention Programs

Programs that seek to prevent youthful drinking/driving and related problems fall into two broad categories, and significant controversy has arisen between the advocates of each.* This section describes each program category and discusses the controversy that surrounds them.

---

*A third category of program comprises those that attempt to reduce the consequences of drinking and driving through making the environment safer. Programs advocating seatbelt use, the installation of airbags, and the use of breakaway road sign posts fall into this category. Such programs are not generally defined as prevention programs, although the similarity of their objectives to those of many other drinking/driving programs (e.g., the reduction of mortality and morbidity) suggests that they probably should be.

The first category of program views drinking/driving as one of a constellation of <u>alcohol-related problems</u> experienced by youth and may thus be termed the "alcohol-related problem strategies." These programs attempt to reduce drinking/driving by reducing the amount of teen drinking using any of the prevention strategies described above. An example of this category of program is "Project Graduation," which provides alcohol-free alternative parties during graduation week, the holiday season, and other similar times.

The second category of program views drinking/driving as one of a constellation of <u>traffic safety problems</u> experienced by youth and may thus be termed the "traffic safety strategies." These programs attempt to reduce drinking/driving by disassociating drinking from driving. Examples of this category of program are "Safe Rides," which provides free, safe transportation to youth who have been drinking or who are with a driver who has been drinking, and the "Contract for Life," in which parents and teens mutually agree to provide a ride home or cab fare if one has been drinking or is with a driver who has been drinking.

As suggested, significant controversy has arisen concerning these two categories of programs. On the one hand, advocates of the alcohol-related problems strategies criticize the traffic safety strategies on the grounds that they may be construed by youth as sanctioning drinking and may also encourage youth to drink by making drinking "safer." Thus, it is argued, although these programs may reduce one alcohol-related problem (e.g., drinking/driving), they may increase the incidence of others (e.g., other accidental trauma or addiction).

On the other hand, advocates of the traffic safety strategies argue that despite the best efforts to prevent youthful drinking, the incidence of such behavior is still significant. Until such time (if ever), it is argued, that youth drinking is eliminated, programs that dissociate drinking and driving are needed to reduce mortality and morbidity.

Interestingly, the controversy between these two positions can be resolved empirically, although the data are not currently available to do so. Specifically, research is needed on whether traffic safety strategies actually do increase teenage drinking, and, if so, by how much. Such data would allow communities to make informed comparisons between the risks (if any) of increased incidence of other alcohol-related problems and the benefits of a decreased incidence of youthful drinking and driving. Until such data are available, communities will have to choose between program alternatives (or choose both alternatives) based on programmatic criteria such as acceptability to adult community members, acceptability to youth, availability of resources, and costs.

SUMMARY

The current armamentarium of drug- and alcohol-prevention strategies is extremely diverse in terms of rationale, risk-factor focus, and institutional location. Although many of these strategies are promising, available evaluation research provides little guidance as to which programs are clearly superior. However, some general guidelines for the practitioner do emerge from the preceding review.

First, the practitioner can support and reinforce the no-drug message that underlies almost all current prevention programs and can reinforce the efforts of youth to find activities and cultivate friends that support a drug-free lifestyle. Moreover, the practitioner can validate factual information concerning the risks of drug and alcohol use when questions are raised by patients and parents.

Second, the practitioner can support community efforts to launch multicomponent prevention programs by promoting the need for a broad-based approach that addresses multiple risk factors. The practitioner can be a particularly powerful spokesperson for the need for programmatic initiatives that involve community change (e.g., restricted availability of alcohol, increased law enforcement) because of his/her natural role as a community leader in health issues.

Finally, the practitioner can help communities and community agencies interpret and evaluate the often confusing popular and scientific prevention literature and can help communities avoid making a large commitment of money or time to a prevention strategy that, while currently popular, may already have been shown to be ineffective.

Chapter 7

ETHICAL AND LEGAL CONSIDERATIONS

INTRODUCTION

In the legally complex world of substance abuse, adolescents exist in a mixed kingdom, afforded some of the protections society offers to children and enjoying some of the rights of adults. The resulting uncertainty creates problems for all social- and health-service providers. It poses particular problems for physicians, who have a specific confidential and private relationship with their patients and, at the same time, have a less specified obligation to their patients' parents.

Two questions are paramount in the minds of many physicians. First, what can a physician do to and for a child without parental consent, given the constraints of law, ethics, and patterns of practice? Second, under what circumstances may a physician act against the wishes of an adolescent; i.e., when is an adolescent out of control or in danger to a degree that trumps the private physician-patient relationship and mandates parent involvement? The following discussion will address these and other related issues.

Children have only been recognized as individuals and afforded special protections and rights since the end of the last century. Before that time, children were generally considered as the property of their parents (more correctly of their fathers), to be worked, schooled, apprenticed, or disciplined (even unto death) as the family authority saw fit or deemed necessary. Children were hanged as pickpockets and punished as adults for the crimes they committed.[1]

This singular lack of official sympathy for the plight, special needs, and undeveloped conscience of the young began to change in the late 1800s with the founding of settlement houses and the passage in Illinois in 1899 of the Family Court Act.[2] This scheme of this first Family Court Act, a form of which was adopted in every other state over the next three decades, established that children had special rights and protections under the law. It presented the then somewhat bizarre notion that children should be held to different moral and legal standards of conduct, tried in private and closed hearings, and punished differently from adults if found guilty of a crime. It reflected the enlightened modern philosophy that moral responsibility evolves with developmental sophistication.

The first Family Court Act defined three categories of problem conduct among children brought under its jurisdiction: delinquent, neglected, and unruly. A delinquent child was one who was found to have committed an act that, if done by an adult, would be a crime. A neglected child was one not properly provided with food, clothing, education, and medical care by his or her parents, although they were financially able to do so. An unruly child (defined also as ungovernable, incorrigible, or otherwise unmanageable in the varying language of state statutes) was one found to oppose the dictates and behavioral expectations of parents or society, although having committed no crime. An example of unruly conduct would be staying out past a parentally imposed curfew or not attending school in violation of compulsory attendance laws. Neither is a crime if done by an adult. Actions falling into this last category, often called "status offenses," have come into disfavor. As a result, the category has been eliminated in some states and is rarely used in others.

Children who are under the legal age for alcohol consumption (now 21 years in the majority of states) and who use alcohol and drugs, may be brought to the attention of the family court under any of the three classifications. They may be charged with delinquent behavior, may be considered neglected, or may be adjudicated unruly.

Despite their origin and their understanding of the needs of children, family courts may present a variety of problems to the adolescent and family. For many families, the

court is a last resort, to be used only when informal net-
works and heartfelt appeals have failed. Some families
hope that a judicial reprimand will provide the force for
change, and sometimes it does—especially when judge,
family, and caregivers can fashion supportive and super-
visory plans. Referral to a family court, however, can also
be frustrating. The family courts are often underfunded
and understaffed, especially in large cities. They are over-
whelmed by the numbers and complexities of the multi-
problem families they deal with, often with inadequate
social service supports. Under such circumstances, a court
referral may help the child but it may also be fruitless. The
family's hopes for support may result only in one more de-
monstration of society's callousness or inability to meet
the needs of poor children and families.

As noted above, the family court was established as a re-
flection of society's judgment that children should not be
held to the same standards of behavior as adults because
they have neither the moral maturity nor the wisdom to
guide independent action. This characterization, and the
consequent need for different treatment, clearly applies to
young children. It becomes less compelling as the child
reaches adolescence and approaches maturity. This judgment has resulted, in recent decades, in the re-entry of adolescents accused of certain types of crimes into the adult
criminal justice system. At present, adolescents are
granted protections and limited in their rights by statute,
by common law, and by decisions of the U.S. Supreme
Court. Many believe that this re-examination of children's
rights began in 1954 with Brown v. the Board of Education,[3] which decreed that black children were protected by
the equal protection clause of the 14th amendment and
were entitled to equality in education. The next landmark
case was In re Gault[4] which held that the "protections" of
the juvenile justice system justify treating a child differently from an adult only if the different treatment truly
benefits the child. Thus, a conviction in a juvenile court
based upon inadequate protections would not stand. In

1969, the Supreme Court held that the right to free speech applied to children and hence protected their right to engage in peaceful political activity and symbolic free speech within the public schools (Tinker v. Des Moines, 1969).[5]

Young women have also been clearly brought under the umbrella of constitutional protections, as evidenced by their right to an abortion. In a series of cases, the Supreme Court held that parents did not have a veto over a minor's choice to abort (Bellotti v. Baird, 1976, 1979; Missouri v. Danforth, 1986).[6,7] Nonetheless, it did find constitutional a state requirement that the parents of a minor planning to have an abortion should be notified by the physician, if possible, and if the child did not offer evidence that she was a mature minor (H.L. v. Matheson, 1981).[8] In addition, the court ruled in 1977 that minors had a right to contraceptive privacy and could not be barred from buying nonprescription contraceptives. The court stated in that case that "rights do not mature magically at adulthood" and that "state restrictions inhibiting privacy rights of minors are valid only if they serve a significant state interest that is not present in the case of an adult" (Carey v. Population Services International, 1977).[9] In summary, special status for children is sometimes justified and independent constitutional rights for children are often protected.

In contrast, in Parham v. J.R. (1979),[10] the Supreme Court held that, given the existence of an appropriate state statute, it was not a violation of a minor's constitutional rights for him/her to be "voluntarily" admitted to a mental institution by his/her parents, even if that minor would not be free to leave the institution thereafter. Moreover, in Wisconsin v. Yoder (1972),[11] the Supreme Court held that it was constitutionally permissible for Amish parents to exclude their children from the public schools, even if this exclusion would seriously hamper later efforts at independent existence.

These cases offer a fair example of Supreme Court decisions that support the independent rights of minors in the context of continued parental control. The message that emerges is ambiguous.

ADOLESCENTS AND HEALTH CARE

Physicians, other health-care providers, and health-care institutions face complex ethical and legal questions when providing health care to adolescents. On the one hand, the adolescent is still a child; on the other, he or she possesses independent rights, especially in matters relating to control of his/her body.

The general rule in regard to children and medical care is that parents have the right to consent to care on behalf of their children but do not have the coequal right to refuse care. Any attempt by a parent to refuse care that is deemed by physicians to be necessary for the health and well-being of a child may and should be referred to the family court as a possible instance of medical neglect. If the court finds medical neglect, it will order treatment despite the parents' opposition. Under these rules, children of Jehovah's Witnesses, for example, are regularly provided blood transfusions, and children of self-healing sects are given chemotherapy for cancer.

When physician and parent agree, parents have the right to consent to care and also to refuse care. In theory, the parent does not refuse in the latter case, but rather the physician does not propose a treatment that he or she believes will not benefit the child and is therefore not in the best interest of that child. In an emergency, care should be provided, even without parental approval, if the child is in pain or if a delay in securing approval might compromise the child's present or future health or well-being.

Parents have the right and responsibility to supervise their child's care because society assumes that the parent's decision will reflect the best interest of the child. The law reflects the well-organized perception that parents are the best advocates for, and protectors of, their child's well-being.

Children, at least young children, do not have the maturity, skill, education, or wisdom to balance present pain against future benefit. For example, a child cannot understand the purpose of a vaccination and the trade-off between present pain and later immunity. Every small child will be deterred merely by the presence of a needle. Children cannot puzzle out complex personal cost-benefit analyses and weigh the risks and benefits that informed consent requires.

Many of the assumptions about children and parents, however, are far from self-evident when the child enters adolescence. By common-law tradition, and in some states by statute, two categories of adolescents can provide consent to care: the mature minor and the emancipated minor. The mature minor is one who, in the subjective judgment of another person, is found to possess the adult cognition and judgment necessary for making health-care decisions. The emancipated minor is one who has joined the armed services, is married, is living apart and financially independent of his or her parents, or otherwise demonstrates clear patterns of independent existence. Mature minors and emancipated minors may consent to their own medical care. Logic would seem to dictate that these two groups be accorded a similar right to refuse care. Such a right, however, is somewhat in doubt, especially if the refusal would have serious, long-lasting health consequences or might lead to death. Another way to think about the mature minor is suggested by an analysis of cases relating specifically to medical care. In that context, the cases demonstrate that a physician has never been found liable for delivering health care to a minor without parental consent and solely on the consent of the minor when:

1) The treatment was undertaken for the benefit of the minor rather than a third party;
2) The minor was near majority (or at least in the range of 15 years of age and up) and was considered to have

sufficient mental capacity to understand fully the nature and importance of the medical steps proposed; and

3) The medical procedures could be characterized by the court as less than "major" or "serious."[12] The doctrine of the mature minor exists in the intersection of a child's ability and the quality of the intervention.

By law, adolescents are therefore similar to but not entirely like small children. There is, needless to say, nothing magical about the age of majority; it is largely a societal convenience. It used to be 21 years of age; however, when the Constitution was amended to lower the voting rights age from 21 to 18 years, most markers of majority followed suit. In addition, many states have enacted "minor treatment statutes" that stipulate ages below 18 (now the age of majority in all states) at which a child can consent to care.[13]

The last two decades have thrown into disarray some assumptions about the relationships of parents and children. Adolescents have become progressively more visible as an independent group within American society, for example, as a sizeable consumer market or as a growing segment of the criminal population. Adolescents' independence and singular lifestyles often reflect a clear distinction of interest between parent and child. For many of these youngsters, who are estranged and alone, it may no longer make sense to require parental involvement in medical care. On the other hand, it could be argued that it is precisely these children who may need a wiser, more mature review of complex decisions.

In recognition of changing lifestyles and sexual mores and in light of the epidemiology of venereal disease and the public health interest in treatment, all states now permit minors to secure medical care and treatment for venereal disease without parental consent.[14] Legislators reasoned that the sensitive nature of the disease and the fear of parental disapproval would discourage young people from seeking care, thus endangering themselves and others. Even if venereal disease treatment were not singled out, providers would likely be protected in providing care without parental consent by the emergency doctrine, given that the dangers of untreated venereal disease are substantial.

The same sort of problem is presented in considering treatment for substance abuse. More than half of the states now have specific statutes permitting treatment for substance abuse without parental consent.[15] In those jurisdictions without specific legislative empowerment, either the emergency doctrine or the emancipated minor category may be applicable. One authority states:

Even in the absence of statute, however, a child with a drug problem who flatly refuses to tell his parents that he needs treatment or to permit the physician to do so undoubtedly would be held competent by a court to give consent to such treatment, since the social and personal consequences to the child of the addiction are so profound and since continuing to make illegal purchases of drugs will subject the child to serious risks of arrest and punishment.[16]

Thus, physicians are not liable for the non-negligent provision of care to a minor without parental consent, in an emergency, if the child is a mature minor or an emancipated minor, or if the care is for venereal disease or substance abuse. Whether the parents could be held financially liable for care to which they have not consented is open to question, and the physician must be ready to absorb the cost of such care. The very attempt to collect from the parent, moreover, could breach the confidential physician-patient relationship.

CONFIDENTIALITY

Confidentiality and protection for the fact of treatment and the conditions of treatment is considered a basic element of health-care delivery and a linchpin of the doctor-patient relationship. All professional oaths for physicians state that it is the physician's ethical obligation to guard the communications of a patient as private and to protect secrets shared between doctor and patient.[17] These oaths are incorporated into most state licensing statutes. In addition, all states, in codification of pre-existing common law, have enacted "privilege statutes" that protect communications between doctor and patient, husband and wife, priest (clergy) and penitent, and lawyer and client. These statutes permit the patient to raise the "privilege" of confidentiality in court in order to exclude otherwise relevant and permissible testimony, especially testimony that may describe the content of the physician-patient interaction. Judges do not favor these statutes, believing that they impede the free flow of otherwise relevant testimony, and therefore tend to construe them narrowly.

Arrayed against these fragile supports for confidentiality are 1) third-party payer contracts that require reports on conditions and treatment, 2) narrow constructions of the legal protections, 3) the computerization of medical information and recordkeeping, and 4) the danger of gossip. In addition, confidentiality is overridden in some circumstances by mandatory reporting laws and in others by the danger to the public or the imminent risk of harm to the patient. Mandatory reporting regulations now require notification of the local health department for a range of illnesses. Venereal disease, for example, must be reported in all states; AIDS in some states. Certain nonreportable behaviors may also require breaching confidentiality and warning a specifically endangered third party. This last exception, called the "Tarasoff rule," (after the California case that established it) requires psychotherapists, and perhaps by extension all physicians, to warn possibly endangered strangers that they may be harmed by a patient (Tarasoff v. The Regents of the State of California, 1976).[18] Such warnings are required if the patient has specifically identified a potential victim, a feasible plan to cause harm and, in the judgment of the therapist, the clear intent to act according to the plan. This ruling originally caused much consternation; however, it has not been followed by many other states. Nonetheless, every local or state medical society should know if the jurisdiction has a so-called "Tarasoff" rule. Moreover, even where warning an endangered third party may not be legally required, a physician may feel morally bound to act.

For the adolescent substance-abuser, issues of confidentiality are even more complex. The basic contract between and among the adolescent, parent (if involved), and physician must acknowledge the possibility of breach from the outset. The physician should make clear to the adolescent or to the parent and adolescent (if they come together) that the statement given and history told by the adolescent and the treatment plan agreed to are confidential and will not be shared with the parent or with any other person, except under certain circumstances. The exceptions are (1) if the patient requests parental involvement, (2) if the patient consents specifically to a parent's request for information, and (3) if the physician concludes that the adolescent's behavior may lead to harm to the patient himself/herself or another person. This contract, shared openly with parent and adolescent, makes all parties knowing participants in the same game played by the same rules.

If an adolescent comes alone to the physician, requests care, and refuses to tell the parent, the physician must decide if he/she is willing to accept the adolescent's consent as a sufficient basis for treatment. This decision is based on the factors discussed previously. Even willing to do so, the physician might stipulate to the minor some limit to confidentiality under an exception relating to direct and immediate harm. A contract regarding confidentiality at the outset provides not only a clear basis for present physician practice but also a guideline for future behavior that should resolve many moral uncertainties.

In general, confidentiality is owed to the adolescent patient because it is that adolescent who stands as the patient in the physician-patient dyad. However, even the most sophisticated and mature adolescent is likely to have areas of less adult behavior, especially if he or she is engaged in self-abusing or self-destructive behavior involving drugs and alcohol.

The Model Act of the American Academy of Pediatrics provides that:

Any minor who has physical or emotional problems and is capable of making rational decisions, and whose relationship with his parents or legal guardian is in such a state that by informing them the minor will fail to seek initial or future help may consent to health professionals for health services...After the professional establishes his rapport with the minor, then he may inform the patient's parents or legal guardian unless such action will jeopardize the life of the patient or the favorable result of the treatment.[19]

There are no well-known cases in which a child has sued a physician for breach of confidentiality because the physician revealed information to a parent or guardian without the child's permission or over the child's objection. There are also no cases in the literature in which a physician was held liable for nondisclosure to a parent when a parent requested information. In contrast to education records, which are specifically available for parent review,[20] medical records remain private and subject to the specific contract and practice exceptions noted above. It would be equally bad practice for a physician to shield a suicidal patient behind a wall of confidentiality or to report an inquisitive but responsible patient who had just become sexually active or had experimented briefly with alcohol. If the sexually active adolescent then became a promiscuous homosexual who did not take appropriate precautions against sexually transmitted disease, or if the adolescent who had taken an initial drink developed a pattern of drunk driving, however, it would no longer be acceptable to guard confidentiality and exclude parents from notice of the potentially destructive or lethal behavior of their child.

Even in these cases, however, the physician should attempt to involve the patient and secure permission for the parental contact. Should all attempts at provider-patient agreement fail, the parent or guardian should be informed.

The physician is never forbidden, either by law or by the application of ethical principles, from sharing information with the parent under circumstances in which the patient is a danger to self or others. In general, the principle of confidentiality is a positive good to be encouraged and supported; it is never an absolute barrier to communication.

If confidentiality were not strongly supported, many fear that adolescents would be less likely to seek continuous care from one health-care provider. If confidentiality were not assured, some adolescents might not seek care at all, while others might seek it in distant localities and provide false histories and incorrect family information, thus making adequate care difficult or impossible.

Some confidential treatment for drug and alcohol abuse is specifically protected by state and federal statutes. More than 35 states and the District of Columbia specifically give juveniles the right to obtain treatment for substance abuse without consent.[21] In addition, there are specific federal Alcohol and Drug Confidentiality Regulations[22] that apply to any program or individual who provides diagnosis, treatment, or referral for alcohol or drug problems and receives federal funds or to any program with a tax-exempt status. These regulations specify that information on a minor patient in such a program can be released only with the patient's prior written and informed release.

Even here, however, where the ethical and legal protections for the patient are strong, they are not absolute. The physician must always be aware that specific planned destructive behavior or self-destructive behavior (suicide) should be considered a potential basis for parental notification.

Physicians should be comfortable about the improbability of liability and the propriety of protecting the patient's secrets when doctrines of confidentiality appear to require excluding the parent from the treatment. The guidelines and specific protections are by now quite clear. But what of the converse? What of a physician asked to screen for substance abuse or requested to treat over the objections of the patient? Screening or treatment over patient objection is a matter for the police power activity of the state; it is not an appropriate activity for medical practitioners.

Two of the inherent powers of government in the Anglo-American tradition are the *parens patriae* power, in which the state intervenes to protect persons not capable of protecting themselves, and the police power, under which the state intervenes to protect others. Both require some formal determination that the individual is not capable of recognizing, defining, and acting responsibly in the pursuit of self-interest and consequently is a possible danger to self or others. Thus, involuntary commitment or involuntary treatment for psychiatric illness requires a petition, argument, and court review. Before an adolescent can be compelled to submit to treatment for substance abuse, some comparable formal process should be required, if argument, persuasion, and cajoling all fail.

It would be practically impossible, and generally inadvisable, for physicians to attempt diagnosis or treatment over the adolescent's objection. The adolescent is the patient; absent his or her consent, diagnosis and treatment cannot and should not proceed. The physician might resort to trickery and take blood or urine samples for one purpose and use them for another. That would be a substantial breach of the trust underlying the doctor-patient relationship.

The parents may seek a court order or the intervention of police in order to impose medical care. Even in these circumstances, however, the physician would not be obligated to comply unless specifically ordered by a judge.

Parents may, as explained at the outset of this comment, seek to have their children found delinquent or unruly so that they may be segregated from society. Once an adolescent is so confined, the medical providers in a juvenile detention setting have the obligation to provide constitutionally adequate care and the right to test within very expanded guidelines. It is unclear, however, if they may impose care without specific court authorization.

If the physician did force care, on parental instructions and over the patient's objection, could he or she be liable later for assault and battery? Answering such a question requires the abilities of a soothsayer, not an attorney. There is no case reported in which a physician has been held liable for care imposed on an adolescent over the patient's objection. Physicians dealing with small children regularly behave in this way. Even the most reasonable two-year-old will resist the pain of inoculation; many must be restrained for treatment that is clearly in their best interest. Older children may have irrational fears of necessary surgery. Some adolescents refuse care based on the oppositional stage of development, not on preference or considered judgment. Thus, there may be limited circumstances in which it is both necessary and appropriate to treat over the objections of a child and, less commonly, over those of the adolescent.

It is more difficult to imagine this analysis applying to treatment for substance abuse. Since alcohol use by a minor is illegal and all drug use is illegal, any adolescent engaged in these behaviors is exhibiting delinquent behavior.[23] If a court so finds, the adolescent may be segregated and ordered to participate in treatment, thus facilitating the coercion of the resistant adolescent.

Diagnosis and treatment of substance abuse is a real and growing problem. Consumption of beer, wine, and hard liquor is rising among teenagers. Drug abuse is increasing and its more virulent forms, such as use of crack and designer drugs, are of special concern. It is not clear that substance abuse is primarily a medical problem. Class, economics, and race, rather than medical care, tend to predict risk. Medicine can be a useful part of a treatment regimen, if accepted and trusted by the patient. Physicians will be more useful as allies of and advocates for, rather than opponents of, the patient's position and wishes.

REFERENCES

1. Aries P: *Centuries of Childhood: A Social History of Family Life.* New York, Vintage Books, 1965
2. Platt AM: *The Child Savers: The Invention of Delinquency.* Chicago, The University of Chicago Press, 1969
3. Brown v. Board of Education, 374 U.S. 483, 1954
4. In re Gault, 387 U.S. 1, 1967
5. Tinker v. Des Moines School District, 393 U.S. 503, 1969
6. Bellotti v. Baird, 424 U.S. 952, 1976; Bellotti v. Baird, 443 U.S. 622, 1979
7. Planned Parenthood of Central Missouri v. Danforth, 428 U.S. 52, 1976
8. H.L. v. Matheson, 450 U.S. 398, 1981
9. Carey v. Population Services International, 431 U.S. 678, 1977
10. Parham v. J.R., 442 U.S. 584, 1979
11. Wisconsin v. Yoder, 406 U.S. 205, 1972
12. Holder AR: *Legal Issues in Pediatrics and Adolescent Medicine.* New Haven, CT, Yale University Press, 1985, p 134
13. Id. at 129
14. Id. at 130
15. Evans DG: *Kids, Drugs & The Law.* United States, Hazelden Foundation, 1985, p 38
16. Holder, supra note 12, at 131
17. Siegler M: Confidentiality & Medicine: A Decrepit Concept. N.E.J.M. 307:1518, 1982
18. Tarasoff v. The Regents of the State of California, 556 P 2d 334, 1976
19. Holder, *supra* note 12 at 143
20. The Federal Family and Educational Rights Privacy Act of 1974, i.e. The Buckley Amendment, 20 USCA Section 1232 g
21. Evans, *supra* note 15, at 37 citing Rosoff
22. Id. at 62
23. Evans, *supra* note 15, at 21

Chapter 8

SPECIFIC DRUGS

INTRODUCTION

This chapter is designed as a reference to assist the primary care practitioner in understanding the pharmacologic, psychoactive, and somatic consequences of particular drugs of abuse. There are literally hundreds of psychoactive drugs that may be abused. This chapter includes only those drugs (or classes of drugs) that are abused by significant numbers of children and adolescents. Presented in order of 30-day prevalence of daily use by adolescents, these drugs include: 1) tobacco; 2) alcohol; 3) marijuana; 4) cocaine; 5) inhalants; 6) stimulants; 7) hallucinogens; 8) phencyclidine (PCP); 9) opiates; 10) sedatives/hypnotics; 11) tranquilizers; and 12) designer drugs.

TOBACCO

1. EPIDEMIOLOGY

Tobacco was smoked or taken as snuff by the natives in North and South America for centuries and was introduced in Europe as a medicinal herb in the sixteenth century.[1] Soon, however, the use of tobacco became a widespread social practice and it remains so today. A significant part of American history revolves around the lucrative tobacco trade from the colonies in Virginia to England. In the nineteenth century, most of the tobacco use by Americans was as chewing tobacco: few people smoked. However, by the "roaring 20s," smoking had taken over chewing and by the 1950s, fueled by the returned veterans of World War II, cigarette smoking became a national habit. As the health dangers of smoking began to be documented and publicized in the 60s and 70s, we began to see a return to the use of chewing or smokeless tobacco.

The smoking behavior of adolescents tends to be similar to that of adults. In general, the prevalence of daily smoking by high school seniors has been decreasing in the last decade, from 27% of youngsters in 1975 to 19% in 1986.[2] A disturbing trend, however, is that adolescent girls now smoke more than boys and constitute one of the few segments of the population where smoking behavior is not decreasing. Twenty percent of senior girls, compared with only 17% of senior boys, were daily smokers in 1986.[2] A household sample survey conducted in Ontario with younger adolescents found that among the 12-13-year-olds, 3% of boys and 4% of girls were regular smokers. Among 14-16-year-olds, 16% of boys and 23% of girls were regular smokers.[3] These data are consistent with those from other studies that indicate initiation of smoking in the early teenage years.

The use of smokeless tobacco is increasing in the adolescent population, particularly among boys. A recent survey of 901 high school students in Arkansas indicated that 37% of boys but only 2% of girls were current users of smokeless tobacco.[4] Similarly, a survey of 609 eighth, ninth, and tenth graders (mean age 14.5 years) in Pittsburgh revealed that 35% of boys and none of the girls reported smokeless tobacco use.[5] In that same survey, 22% of girls but only 11% of boys reported smoking cigarettes.

The Childhood Antecedents of Smoking Study (CASS), a prospective longitudinal investigation conducted in Minnesota, documented predictors of smoking behavior among young adolescents who had not yet become regular smokers.[6] These included: peer influence (having friends who smoke), having siblings who smoke, having less educated parents (especially for girls), being more independent and rebellious, and being less concerned about the health consequences of smoking. This latter finding was considered encouraging by the authors because it suggests that for younger adolescents "there may yet be value in communicating messages about the health consequences of smoking." A recent retrospective study examining the cognitive and school performance characteristics preceding the onset of smoking in high school students found that cigarette smoking in high school was associated with significantly more school absence in elementary school as well as in high school, lower grade point averages in grades four and six as well as in high school, lower I.Q. in sixth grade, and lower scores on Stanford Achievement Tests in both third and fifth grades.[7] These associations suggest that smoking behavior may be part of lifestyle differences among children and adolescents and that smoking prevention efforts must begin early and "address general values and lifestyles rather than only the practice of smoking."

2. CLINICAL PHARMACOLOGY

The active ingredient of cigarette smoke and chewed or snorted tobacco is nicotine.[1] This is a naturally occurring alkaloid that is well absorbed in the lungs by inhalation or through the mucous membranes of the mouth and nose. Nicotine is deactivated in the liver and excreted by the kidneys. Tolerance develops with continued use, at least partially because of increased activity of the liver microsomal enzyme systems responsible for deactivation of the drug. Nicotine appears to play a central role in the dependence-producing process of cigarette smoking; however, to claim that smoking is primarily a nicotine addiction would be to ignore the very powerful roles of environmental and social influences and learning behavior that contribute to the initiation and perpetuation of tobacco use.

In the peripheral nervous system, nicotine blocks cholinergic synapses and also has a sympathomimetic effect via stimulation of the release of adrenaline. Nicotine is highly toxic. Symptoms of low-level poisoning—dizziness, nausea, and generalized weakness—are frequently noticed by beginning smokers. A toxic overdose can lead to tremors, convulsions, paralysis of the respiratory muscles, and death. In the central nervous system, nicotine acts to shift the electroencephalogram into an arousal pattern.

However, most smokers claim that the net effect is relaxation and relief of tension.

Other components of cigarette smoke play a key role in the toxicity of smoking. Carbon monoxide is one such component. Regular smokers have a higher-than-normal amount of carboxy-hemoglobin, which impairs the oxygen-carrying capacity of their blood. This often contributes to dyspnea on exertion in smokers and impairs oxygen transfer to the fetus via the placenta in pregnant women who smoke. Tars and other carcinogens in both smokeless tobacco and cigarette smoke are responsible for the association between tobacco use and malignancies.

3. HEALTH CONSEQUENCES

The contribution of cigarette smoking to excess morbidity and mortality from heart disease, emphysema, and lung cancer in older Americans is well known and will not be restated here.[8] Instead, the focus will be on the health consequences of smoking and tobacco use for the pediatric patient: the fetus, neonate, infant, child, and adolescent.

The fetus of the smoking mother suffers from chronic hypoxia; the result is generalized growth retardation marked by decreases in birth weight, length, and circumference of the head, chest, and shoulders.[8] In addition, the fetus of a woman who smokes is at increased risk of preterm delivery. Because of these varied adverse effects, the neonate of a smoking mother is at increased risk for death.[8]

Infants and young children of smoking parents are at increased risk for serious respiratory illnesses such as bronchitis and pneumonia. One study found that children whose mothers smoked had a hospital admission rate for respiratory illness that was 28% higher than that of children of nonsmoking mothers.[8] Other studies have documented that asthma, persistent middle-ear effusions, and sudden infant death are all more common in children of smokers than of nonsmokers.[8] While these statistical associations do not prove cause and effect, the evidence that passive smoking impairs the health of children is compelling. Significantly increased amounts of nicotine and its metabolite, cotinine, have been measured in the urine and saliva of infants less than one year of age who were exposed to parental tobacco smoke.[9] This provides definite evidence that these infants do passively absorb the constituents of smoke from their environment.

A number of studies have found measurable impairment of small, peripheral airway function in adolescent smokers. One longitudinal study in Boston documented a significant decline in forced expiratory volume in one second (FEV_1) and in the middle half of forced vital capacity (FVC) in adolescents who became smokers compared with their nonsmoking peers.[10] The pulmonary function parameters of these children were not different from those of their peers before the onset of smoking. The Berlin-Breman study of seventh and eighth graders documented a linear decline in the ratio of FEV_1 to FVC as carbon monoxide levels in expired air (a measure of recent smoking) increased.[11] This study also showed an inverse relationship between smoking in adolescents and high-density lipoprotein-cholesterol (HDL-C) that was evident within two years of beginning to smoke. Thus, data are accumulating to suggest that abnormalities known to be precursors of smoking-related disease are measurable in young people within a few years of initiation of the behavior.

4. LABORATORY EVALUATION

Methods commonly used to verify smoking behavior include measuring saliva or urinary cotinine and nicotine concentrations, carboxyhemoglobin or thiocyanate concentration in blood, and concentrations of carbon monoxide in expired air. These measures are used primarily in research studies.

5. TREATMENT

The most effective treatment for cigarette smoking is to prevent the onset of the behavior. This is particularly important in the child and young adolescent. The most successful smoking-prevention programs are school-based, target the very early adolescent in sixth or seventh grade, use peer counselors, emphasize positive health behaviors rather than dwelling on risks, discuss risks that are immediate and applicable to the age group, and teach skills for resisting the social pressures to smoke.[12,13] Pediatricians have a significant role to play in seizing every opportunity to discourage smoking among the parents of their infant and child patients and especially among their adolescent patients.[14,15] Particular attention should be addressed to teenaged girls. There are data indicating that physician counseling regarding the hazards of tobacco use is effective, even if it only occurs at one visit. For adolescents who are already smokers and wish to quit, there are myriad smoking-cessation programs of variable effectiveness. Nicotine gum may be helpful as an adjunct to treatment.[16] Many smokers try to quit several times before they eventually succeed; thus, the message should be to keep trying. In addition, curtailment of tobacco advertisers, who deliberately target women (including adolescent women) in their advertisements, may be necessary.

REFERENCES

1. Ray O: *Drugs, Society, and Human Behavior.* 3rd edition. St. Louis, C.V. Mosby Co., 1983; pp 183-205
2. Johnston LD, O'Malley PM, Bachman JG: *Drug Use by High School Seniors—The Class of 1986,* US Department of Health and Human Services publication No. (ADM) 87-1535. Rockville, MD,1987
3. Boyle MH, Offord DR: Smoking, drinking and use of illicit drugs among adolescents in Ontario: prevalence, patterns of use and sociodemographic correlates. *Can Med Assoc J* 1986; 135:1113-1121
4. Manty PJ, McDermott RJ, Williams T: Patterns of smokeless tobacco use in a population of high school students. *Am J Pub Health* 1986; 76(2):190-192
5. Guggenheimer J, Zullo TG, et al: Changing trends of tobacco use in a teenage population in western Pennsylvania. *Am J Pub Health* 1986; 76(2):196-197
6. Mittlemark MB, Murray DM, Luepker RV, et al: Predicting experimentation with cigarettes: The Childhood Antecents of Smoking Study (CASS). *Am J Pub Health* 1987; 77(2):206-208

7. Young TL, Rogers KD: School performance characteristics preceding onset of smoking in high school students. *Am J Dis Child* 1986; 140:257-259
8. Fielding JE: Smoking: health effects and control. Part 1. *N Engl J Med* 1985; 313(8):491-498
9. Greenberg RA, Haley NJ, Etzel RA, et al: Measuring the exposure of infants to tobacco smoke. *N Engl J Med* 1984;310(17):1075-1078
10. Tager IB, Munoz A, Rosner B, et al: Effect of cigarette smoking on the pulmonary function of children and adolescents. *Am Rev Respir Dis* 1985; 131:752-759
11. Dwyer JH, Lippert P, Rieger-Ndakorerwa GE, et al: Some chronic disease risk factors and cigarette smoking in adolescents: the Berlin-Bremen study. *MMWR Supplement* 1987;36(45):355-405
12. Perry CL, Killen J, Telch M, et al: Modifying smoking behavior of teenagers: a school based intervention. *Am J Pub Health* 1980; 70(7):722-725
13. Schinke SP, Gilchrist LD, Snow WH: Skills intervention to prevent cigarette smoking among adolescents. *Am J Pub Health 985; 75(6):665-667*
14. Perry CL, Silvis GL: Smoking prevention: behavioral prescriptions for the pediatrician. *Pediatrics* 1987; 79(5):790-799
15. Committee on Adolescence, American Academy of Pediatrics: Tobacco use by childen and adolescents. *Pediatrics* 1987;79(3):479-481
16. Blum A: Nicotine chewing gum and the medicalization of smoking. *Ann Intern Med* 1984; 101(1):121-123

ALCOHOL

1. EPIDEMIOLOGY

Aside from caffeine, alcohol is used by more people and in larger quantities than any other psychoactive substance. Alcoholic beverages have been consumed by humans since the dawn of time (neolithic man drank berry wine in 6400 B.C.), and efforts to regulate consumption have gone on for centuries. In 1839, England imposed penalties for selling spirits to persons under the age of 16 years, while in the various states of this country, the legal drinking age continues to fluctuate between 18 and 21 years. Despite efforts to regulate teenage drinkers, enormous numbers of adolescents consume alcohol. In 1986, 91% of American high school seniors had tried alcohol, 65% had consumed it within the past month, and 5% drank alcohol daily. In the past, men were more likely to drink than women, but at least in the adolescent population, these differences seem to be lessening. Among high school seniors in 1986, 69% of males and 61% of females reported alcohol use in the past month.[2] Boys were still more likely to be very frequent drinkers, with 7%, versus only 3% of girls, reporting daily alcohol use. Data from a Canadian household sample survey conducted in 1983 found that among younger adolescents, girls reported more alcohol use than boys: 49% of girls versus 43% of boys were occasional alcohol drinkers, and 16% of girls but only 11% of boys in this cohort of 14-16-year-olds reported using alcohol once a week or more.

Children of alcoholic parents are more likely to become alcoholics themselves. It is widely acknowledged that there is some genetic component to alcoholism, especially for men (See Chapter 1). In addition, family life with an alcoholic parent is often disruptive and sometimes abusive and can lead to a wide variety of problem behaviors in adolescent children, including alcohol and drug abuse.

2. PHARMACOLOGY

Ethyl alcohol (C2H5OH) is produced by fermentation of the starch or sugar in various fruits and grains by the action of yeast. Fermentation alone will not produce a beverage with greater than 15% alcohol because the yeast dies at higher concentrations. More potent alcoholic products must be produced by distillation from the fermented mash. Alcohol is consumed in the form of beer, made from barley and hops and containing approximately 5% alcohol; wine, made from grapes, approximately 15% alcohol; and spirits or "hard liquor" (scotch, rum, vodka, gin), distilled from barley, corn, or sugar cane, approximately 45% alcohol.

Alcohol is quickly and efficiently absorbed from the gastrointestinal tract and requires no digestion.[1] The rate of absorption depends on the concentration of alcohol, the amount and type of food in the stomach, and whether or not the liquid is carbonated. Diluted alcohol is absorbed more slowly than a highly concentrated "shot" of liquor. However, if the diluent is carbonated or the alcoholic product itself is effervescent (e.g., champagne) it will pass more rapidly into the small bowel and be absorbed even faster than in the stomach. Eating foods containing fat and/or protein before or while drinking alcohol will help to delay absorption.

Drug effects are noticed approximately 10 minutes after consumption and peak at approximately 40-60 minutes after ingestion. In order to be excreted, alcohol must first be oxidized in the liver by the enzyme alcohol dehydrogenase.[4] The activity of this enzyme, not the concentration of alcohol in the blood, is the rate-limiting step in alcohol excretion. Since alcohol cannot be stored in the body and very little can be excreted by the lungs or kidneys, it will remain in the bloodstream unchanged until metabolized by the liver. If an individual consumes alcohol at a faster rate than it can be metabolized, the blood alcohol concentration will rise. The initial metabolic product is acetaldehyde, a compound that may play a central role in alcohol toxicity.

Tolerance to alcohol develops with frequent moderate-to- heavy consumption. Some of this tolerance can be explained by the induction of enzymes in the liver, which allows faster metabolism of the drug, and some by brain tolerance, an adaptation to the neuropsychological effects of alcohol.[5] Physical dependence develops after years of heavy consumption, after which abstinence can result in delirium tremens, a withdrawal syndrome that can lead to seizures and death. This serious withdrawal syndrome has not been described in an adolescent.

3. HEALTH CONSEQUENCES

Alcohol is a central nervous system depressant. At high blood levels, it leads to respiratory depression, arrest, and death. At low blood levels, alcohol impairs regulatory and inhibitory control mechanisms in the brain. Complex and poorly learned behaviors, such as driving in young people, are impaired. Individuals often become generally disinhibited and engage in behaviors that would ordinarily embarrass them. Anxiety is reduced; judgment is poor; and attention, short-term memory, and thought processing are impaired. As blood alcohol levels rise, motor coordination becomes impaired, and reaction time becomes quite prolonged. If drinking continues, stupor, coma, and death can ensue.

For the majority of adolescents, the adverse physical health consequences of alcohol consumption result primarily from accidental trauma incurred while intoxicated.[5] Alcohol-related motor vehicle accidents are the leading cause of death for 15-24-year-old Americans either as drivers or passengers. Other types of accidents such as drownings, falls, or fire-related deaths in adolescents have also been shown to be frequently associated with alcohol intoxication.[6] In addition, elevated blood alcohol levels are found in a significant percentage of adolescent suicide and homicide victims. Physical complications of acute intoxication such as coma, gastrointestinal bleeding, aspiration pneumonia, or acute pancreatitis are relatively rare in teenagers, and are usually the result of the ingestion of a large quantity of alcohol over a short period of time. Complications of chronic alcoholism such as cirrhosis of the liver or Wernike's encephalopathy are virtually unknown in adolescents.

Psychosocial and emotional problems are frequently associated with alcohol use by teenagers. It is often difficult to differentiate whether this emotional ill health is a cause or an effect of the alcohol use. One study of 171 acutely intoxicated 12-18-year-olds brought to the emergency room of a large hospital found that alcohol intoxication was the predominant initial problem in 88% of these young persons.[7] Extensive psychosocial investigation of these teenagers and their families led to the conclusion that alcohol or another drug was the primary problem in 41% of these youth. Nineteen percent were judged to have a primary emotional or psychological problem, 17% had a family problem, 3% had peer relation problems, and 20% had no serious psychosocial problems. Of the 171 intoxicated adolescents, 28% had alcohol-dependent fathers.

Since alcohol use by teenagers is so prevalent, it is important to define alcohol abuse in this age group. Relatively few—less than 5%—of adolescents could be considered alcoholics, that is, addicted to alcohol. Those teenagers who drink daily, have a family history of alcoholism, have blackouts or withdrawal symptoms, and continue drinking despite many negative family, school, and social consequences may be considered to be alcoholics. A much larger group of adolescents, however, may be considered problem drinkers.[8] Fully 19% of 14-17-year-olds fall into this category.[6] These are young people who have been drunk six or more times per year and/or who experience negative consequences from alcohol use two or more times a year.[8] The negative consequences include driving after drinking and troubles with family, friends, teachers, police, or dates because of drinking. Teenage problem drinkers are at especially high risk for accidents and for significant developmental, educational, and emotional difficulties. Finally, adolescents who are neither alcoholics nor problem drinkers but who nevertheless occasionally drink and become intoxicated are still at some risk for accidents and acute overdose.

Alcohol is a known teratogen and appears to have its greatest effect on the developing fetus if consumed in large doses early in pregnancy.[9] Many sexually active adolescent girls fail to use adequate contraception, and unintended, undiagnosed pregnancy is endemic in this age group. Thus, many fetuses of adolescent girls are exposed to the harmful effects of alcohol as well as to the secondary additive effects of poor nutrition and multiple drug abuse.

4. LABORATORY EVALUATION

Behavioral effects and alcohol toxicity correlate well with blood alcohol levels, which are expressed as grams of alcohol per 100 milliliters of blood. A blood alcohol level of 0.05% is usually associated with a "high" feeling; a level of 0.20% is associated with marked intoxication; at 0.30%, the individual is usually stuporous; and death can occur at blood alcohol levels beginning at 0.35%. The concentration of alcohol in the breath is directly related to blood alcohol levels and this fact is used by law enforcement agencies as a noninvasive method for determining blood alcohol levels. Most agencies define alcohol intoxication as a blood alcohol level of 0.10% or higher. Among 16-19-year-olds who had been drinking and were involved in fatal motor vehicle accidents in 1982, blood alcohol levels of 0.10%-0.14% occurred most frequently.[10] Only 16% of the adolescents had levels less than 0.10% and 28% had levels above 0.14%.

5. TREATMENT CONSIDERATIONS

Acute intoxication should be treated with protective and supportive therapy, including maintenance of the airway and respiratory support with a ventilator, if necessary, until the alcohol can be metabolized and the patient recovers. Large overdoses may cause hypoglycemia, particularly in children, and blood glucose levels should be monitored. When present, hypoglycemia should be corrected rapidly by administering an intravenous glucose solution.

Adolescents who might be considered alcoholics, either by psychosocial criteria or, in rare instances, by physiologic addiction, may require treatment in a residential treatment facility staffed by individuals with experience and training in the management of adolescent drug abuse. Disulfiram (Antabuse®), a drug that causes headache, nausea, vomiting and vertigo when alcohol is consumed, may be a useful adjunct to the treatment of the adolescent alcoholic.[12] For the large numbers of adolescents who are problem drinkers, community programs, peer support groups, and individual and family counseling by mental health professionals can all be helpful. Community-based programs, such as Alcoholics Anonymous, that have a history of success in treating adults are less commonly used by young people, who may find little in common with the majority of older group members. Programs specific to young people (e.g., Alateen) are available in some communities.

REFERENCES

1. Ray O: *Drugs, Society and Human Behavior.* 3rd edition. St. Louis, C.V. Mosby Co., 1983, pp145-182
2. Johnston LD, O'Malley PM and Bachman JG: *Drug Use by High School Seniors - The Class of 1986,* US Department of Health and Human Services publication No.(ADM) 87-1535. Rockville, MD, 1987
3. Boyle MH, Offord DR: Smoking, drinking and use of illicit drugs among adolescents in Ontario: prevalence patterns of use and sociodemographic correlates. *Can Med Assoc J* 1986; 135:1113-1121
4. Lieber CS: The metabolism of alcohol. *Sci Am* 1976; 234(3):3-11
5. Committee on Adolescence, American Academy of Pediatrics. Alcohol use and abuse: a pediatric concern. *Pediatrics* 1987; 79(3):450-453
6. Friedman IM: Alcohol and unnatural deaths in San Francisco youths. *Pediatrics* 1985; 76(2):191-193
7. Stephenson JN, Moberg MA, Daniels BJ, et al: Treating the intoxicated adolescent. *JAMA* 1984; 252:1884-1888
8. Donovan JE, Jessor R: Adolescent problem drinking. *J Stud Alcohol* 1978; 39(9):1506-1524
9. Ouelette EM, Rosett HL, Rosman NP, et al: Adverse effects on offspring of maternal alcohol abuse during pregnancy. *N Engl J Med* 1977; 297:528-530
10. Anon: Blood alcohol concentrations among young drivers - United States, 1982. *MMWR* 1983; 32(49):646-648
11. Lovejoy FH: Ethanol Intoxication. *Clin Toxicol Rev* 1981; Vol. 4, No. 2
12. Frank M, Lovejoy FH: Disulfiram. *Clin Toxicol Rev* 1984; Vol. 6, No. 11

MARIJUANA

1. EPIDEMIOLOGY

Over 50 million Americans have tried marijuana. Among high school seniors in the United States, over half have used the drug at least once in their lifetime with approximately 40% reporting use within the last year, making marijuana the most common illicit drug chosen by adolescents.[1] With the exception of cigarettes, marijuana is the substance chosen most often by young people for regular use: 4% of high school seniors use it daily. A national survey in Canada demonstrated that almost 17% of adolescents between the ages of 12 and 19 years had used marijuana within the past year and that 1% used it daily.[2]

2. PHARMACOLOGY

Marijuana is obtained from the hemp plant (Cannabis sativa). The pharmacological effects are related to the content of delta-9-tetrahydrocannabinol (THC) and other cannabinoids that are found in the leaves and flowering shoots. A resinous exudate called hashish, which is derived from the tops of female plants, contains the greatest concentration of active material. THC is the constituent primarily responsible for the neurophysiological, biochemical, and behavioral manifestations of marijuana. Its concentration, and accordingly, the dose delivered may vary by as much as a hundredfold, depending on such factors as the presence of contaminants and diluents. Awareness of this variation in potency is essential when comparing studies of the effects of marijuana as well as in managing the intoxicated patient.

Effects begin within seconds to minutes after inhalation of the smoke or within 30 to 60 minutes following oral ingestion. Smoking routes the cannabinoids directly from the lungs to the brain and other organs, with minimal opportunity for dilution or metabolism. Thus, higher concentrations are delivered to the brain more rapidly when marijuana is inhaled than when it is ingested orally or injected intravenously. While the smoker experiences the effects almost immediately and can stop further inhalation at any time, the oral user experiences effects that come on more slowly, last longer, and are more variable, making unpleasant reactions more likely. Although the initially high blood levels of THC fall rapidly over the first 30 minutes, further elimination occurs more slowly. It takes approximately 19 hours for one half of the initial level to disappear.[3] While repeated use results in an accumulation of cannabinoids, blood levels do not accurately reflect concentrations present in the brain or other organs because the cannabinoids are readily distributed into tissues throughout the body. This is quite different from alcohol, where blood levels do accurately represent those concurrently found in the brain. It also differs from other psychoactive drugs such as caffeine, and nicotine, which are rapidly metabolized and completely eliminated, thereby making detection impossible only a few hours after intake.

3. HEALTH CONSEQUENCES

Although the major effects of marijuana are on behavior, the use of this drug is not without physiologic and somatic consequences.

The acute cardiovascular effects of marijuana include transient increases in heart rate and blood pressure, although mild orthostatic hypotension may also occur. These effects, most likely attributable to THC-induced changes of autonomic function, are temporary and have no deleterious effects in the normal individual. However, it is theoretically possible that adverse consequences may occur in individuals with pre-existing cardiac abnormalities such as atherosclerotic disease of the coronary arteries or congestive heart failure. Long-term users of marijuana may experience sodium retention and an expanded plasma volume,[4] but data regarding adverse clinical effects related to these changes are lacking.

In normal or asthmatic individuals, the immediate pulmonary effect of inhalation of marijuana smoke is bronchodilation.[5,6] For some smokers, however, the particles in the inhalant act as an irritant, causing bronchoconstriction. Furthermore, in chronic users, airway obstruction, as measured by a reduced forced expiratory volume in one second (FEV_1), does occur.[7] Pharyngitis, sinusitis, bronchitis, and asthma have been reported in heavy smokers, particularly hashish users. There is recent evidence that smoking marijuana results in much higher carbon monoxide levels in the blood and tar deposition in the lung than use of a similar quantity of tobacco.[8] Unfortunately, most studies that have attempted to examine the long-term effects of marijuana use in humans have been confounded by the fact that the subjects being investigated also smoke tobacco cigarettes. Data regarding neoplastic potential are inconclusive, but the presence of carcinogens in marijuana smoke and epithelial abnormalities known to be the precursors of lung cancer in tobacco users make this an important subject for future study.[9,10,11]

Concern regarding the impact of marijuana on fertility, arising from studies of men who are heavy users, demonstrate diminished sperm motility and decreased sperm counts, both reversible effects.[12] Animal data show that marijuana interferes with ovulation and causes a decrease in circulating pituitary gonadotropins.[13] However, no evidence exists to directly implicate marijuana as an etiologic factor in infertility in humans.

There remains some question as to whether long-term use of marijuana may suppress cellular-mediated immunity, as measured by reduced lymphocytes. Some animal and human studies have suggested that circulating immunoglobulins are diminished in marijuana users.[14] This raises the possibility that the changes induced and observed in the laboratory may result in lowered resistance to disease in the clinical setting.

The most clearly established effects of marijuana are behavioral changes, which are mediated through the central nervous system. Although earlier studies suggested that brain atrophy may be induced by marijuana, this research was later found to be methodologically flawed. Data from computer tomography indicate no gross morphological changes in the brain. Animal studies on microscopic changes are inconclusive.

Marijuana does induce neurochemical changes in the brain; however, these do not appear to have any deleterious neurologic outcome. Although a temporary effect on brain neurotransmitters has been demonstrated, no long-term toxic effects on production of these neurotransmitters has been observed. The effects of the drug upon brain electrical activity, as measured by electroencephalogram, occur acutely during use, but disappear with discontinuation of the drug. They probably have no effect on susceptibility to epileptic seizures.[15]

The major deleterious effects of marijuana are behavioral rather than somatic. The extent of behavioral effects is usually directly related to the concentration of marijuana used, although the personality of the user, his or her expectation of the effect, and the milieu in which the drug is used also have a contributing role. The popularity of marijuana arises from the euphoria, sense of relaxation, and increased visual, auditory, and taste perceptions it produces in most young people in low or moderate doses. Unpleasant effects may occur with larger doses. These dysphoric reactions tend to occur more often in adults, especially the elderly, but they can occur at any age, particularly in novice users and when intoxication occurs unexpectedly. These dysphoric reactions range from mild fear to distortions in body image, depersonalization, disorientation, and even paranoia and acute panic reactions. Although delirium and hallucinations have also been reported, these extreme reactions should raise suspicion that phencyclidine has been mixed with the marijuana, an event that often occurs without the user's knowledge.

Marijuana has a major effect on performance of tasks related to coordination. Lack of hand steadiness, decreased postural stability manifested by an increase in body sway, and an inaccuracy in the execution of various movements are observed with doses commonly used in social settings. The capacity to follow a moving object (tracking) is adversely effected by even very low doses and may persist after the sensation of intoxication has passed. Studies, still inconclusive, have demonstrated an increase in reaction time and a diminished ability to detect a brief flash of light, effects that may in part be due to a lack of sustained attention.[16] Time perception is altered so that subjects under the influence of moderate doses of the drug consistently overestimate the amount of time that has elapsed.[17] Even minor impairment in tracking ability, reaction time, time sense and visual perceptual functioning have obvious and important implications for everyday situations such as driving an automobile or operating complicated machinery.

Marijuana also seems to exert a major effect on learning and memory. Short-term memory, especially when it is heavily dependent on attention, such as during information acquisition and storage, is significantly affected even by a single moderate dose.[18] Problem-solving skills that are acquired while using the drug are reduced, learning takes place more slowly, and "state-dependent" learning occurs.[19] The latter phenomenon is an interesting situation wherein material that is learned while under the influence of the drug is best remembered in the state of drug intoxication in which it was originally learned. Even though information acquisition does occur, the quality of the learning experience is diminished because the data or skills learned in the drug-intoxicated state are reduced or impaired.

Individuals under the influence of marijuana have trouble organizing their thoughts and stories, utter shorter phrases, speak more slowly, and use irrelevant words in their conversation. These factors have an obvious negative effect on oral dialogue.

An "acute brain syndrome," or delirium, may occur in chronic, heavy users of marijuana.[20] It includes an impairment in ability to sustain attention to environmental stimuli and to maintain goal-directed thinking or behavior, memory or orientation impairment, perceptual disturbances, and changes in sleep pattern, psychomotor activity, or both. The symptom complex unfolds over a brief period of time and fluctuates rapidly. It disappears between several days to several weeks after discontinuation of the drug.

The "amotivational syndrome" consists of loss of energy, apathy, absence of ambition, loss of effectiveness, inability to carry out long-term plans, problems with concentrating, impaired memory, and a marked decline in school or work performance.[21,22] The evidence for an etiologic relationship between marijuana and the amotivational syndrome remains equivocal, as evidence is available only from case reports and similar symptoms are seen in individuals who have not used marijuana.[23] Furthermore, many troubled individuals use drugs as a way to escape from their problems; thus, marijuana use may be a result of pre-existing behavioral problems rather than the cause.

"Flashbacks," a hallucinatory phenomenon that has been consistently described but is without a pharmacological explanation, seem to occur in some users of marijuana. However, most individuals who experience them have a prior history of LSD use and it is probable that the marijuana precipitates LSD flashbacks.[24]

Marijuana produces pharmacologic tolerance after several days of regular use; thus, it is not surprising that a clinical withdrawal syndrome occurs with discontinuation of the drug. Symptoms, which are in the main restricted to chronic users, include irritability, agitation, insomnia, and electroencephalographic changes. They peak at 30 hours after marijuana has been discontinued and disappear without specific therapy within three to four days.[25]

The only objective sign of intoxication with marijuana is conjunctival injection, although noted previously, there may be mild tachycardia and orthostatic hypotension. The clinical diagnosis of marijuana intoxication is based upon a constellation of behavioral symptoms, and is confirmed by history or laboratory evaluation.

Although delta-9-THC crosses the placenta and, when given in high dosages, has been shown to be teratogenic and to induce growth retardation in animals, studies in humans are flawed by confounding factors such as concomitant use of other drugs and are thus, at this time, inconclusive.[26]

4. LABORATORY EVALUATION

Blood testing is available and plasma levels do correlate with the individual's degree of exposure. Marijuana and its metabolites may be detected in the urine within an hour after the drug has been smoked; however, results from urine testing may be quite variable and subject to misinterpretation. For an infrequent user, the test will usually remain positive for several days. Metabolites may be stored in adipose tissue of heavy users, and a urine assay in these individuals may be positive as much as one month after cessation of use (See Chapter 4).

5. TREATMENT CONSIDERATIONS

There is no specific treatment recommended for acute reactions to marijuana other than reassurance for individuals who become anxious or undergo a panic reaction. Talking to these people in a calm, nonthreatening manner in a tranquil milieu can often be quite helpful.

REFERENCES

1. Johnston LD, O'Malley PM, Bachman JG: *Drug Use by High School Seniors - The Class of 1986,* US Department of Health and Human Services publication No.(ADM) 87-1535. Rockville, MD, 1987
2. Anon.: Trends in self-reported marijuana use among teenagers-Canada, 1981-1983. *MMWR* 1984; 33(43):609
3. Hunt A, Jones RT: Tolerance and disposition of tetra-hydrocannabinol in man. *J Pharmacol Exp Ther* 1980; 215:35-44

4. Benowitz NL, Jones RT: Cardiovascular effects of prolonged delta-9-tetrahydrocannabinol ingestion. *Clin Pharmacol Ther* 1975; 22:259-297

5. Vachon L, Fitzgerald MX, Solliday NH, et al: Single-dose effect of marihuana smoke: bronchial dynamics and respiratory-center sensitivity in normal subjects. *N Engl J Med* 1973;288:985-989,

6. Tashkin DP, Shapiro BJ, Frank IM: Acute pulmonary physiologic effects of smoked marijuana and oral delta-9-tetrahydrocannabinol in healthy young men. *N Engl J Med* 1973;289:336-341

7. Tashkin DP, Calvarese BM, Simmons MS, et al: Respiratory status of seventy-four habitual marijuana smokers. *Chest* 1980;78:699-706

8. Wu TC, Tashkin DP, Djahed B, et al: Pulmonary hazards of smoking marijuana as compared with tobacco. *N Engl J Med* 1988;318:347-351

9. Busch FW, Seid DA, Wei, ET: Mutagenic activity of marijuana smoke condensates. *Cancer Lett* 1979; 6:319-324

10. Novotny M, Lee ML, Bartle KD: A possible chemical basis for the high mutagenicity of marijuana smoke as compared to tobacco smoke. *Experientia* 1976; 32:280-282

11. Tenant FS, Preble M, Prendergast TJ, et al: Medical manifestations associated with hashish. *JAMA* 1971; 219:1965-1969

12. Hembree WC, Nahas GG, Zeidenberg P, et al: Changes in human spermatozoa associated with high dose marijuana smoking, in Nahas GG, Paton WDM (eds): *Marijuana: Bilogical Effects, Analysis, Metabolism, Cellular Responses, Reproduction and Brain*. Oxford, England, Pergamon Press, 1979; pp 424-439

13. Asch RH, Smith CG, Siler-Khodr TM, et al: Effects of delta-9-tetrahydrocannabinol during the follicular phase of the rhesus monkey. *J Clin Endocrinol Metab* 1981; 52:50-55

14. American Medical Association, Council on Scientific Affairs: Marijuana: its health hazards and therapeutic potentials. *JAMA* 1981; 246:1823-1827

15. Karler R, Turkanis SA: The cannabinoids as potential antiepileptics. *J Clin Pharmacol* 1981; 21(suppl):4375

16. National Research Council, Institute of Medicine, Division of Health Science Policy: Behavioral and psychosocial effects of marijuana use, in Relman A(ed): *Marijuana and Health*, Washington,D.C., National Academy Press, 1982; pp 112-138

17. Milstein SL, MacCannell K, Karr G, et al: Marijuana produced impairments of coordination. *J Nerv Ment Dis* 1975; 161:26-31

18. Abel EL: Marijuana and memory. *Nature* 1970; 227:1151-1152

19. Darley CF, Tinklenberg JR, Roth WT, et al: Marijuana effects on long-term memory assessment and retrieval. *Psychopharmacology* 1977; 53:239-241

20. Meyer RE: Psychiatric consequences of marijuana use: The state of the evidence, in Tinklenberg, JR (ed): *Marijuana and Health Hazards: Methodological Issues in Current Research*, NewYork, Academic Press, 1975; pp 133-152

21. McGlothlin WH, West LJ: The marijuana problem: An overview.*Am J Psychiatry* 1968; 125:370-378

22. Thurlow HJ: On drive state and cannabis: A clinical observation. *Can Psychiatr Assoc J* 1971; 16:181-182

23. Brill NQ, Christie RL: Marijuana and psychosocial adaptation. *Arch Gen Psychiatry* 1974; 31:713-719

24. Stanton MD, Mintz J, Franklin RM: Drug flashbacks II. Some additional findings. *Int J Addict* 1976; 11:53-69

25. Jones RT, Benowitz N: The 30-day trip - clinical studies of cannabis tolerance and dependence, in Braude MC and Szara S(eds): *Pharmacology of Marihuana*, New York, Raven Press, 1976; pp 627-642

26. Abel EL: Prenatal exposure to cannabis: A critical review of effects on growth, development, and behavior. *Behav Neural Biol*1980; 29:137-156

COCAINE

1. EPIDEMIOLOGY

Cocaine use by adolescents has increased dramatically in recent years. National surveys of high school seniors show that cocaine use increased from 9% in the class of 1975 to 17.3% in the class of 1986.[1] The increase in adolescent cocaine use is occurring among males and females, among college-bound and non-college-bound students, and among teenagers in many different geographic areas.

The growing popularity of cocaine use among adolescents can be attributed to a combination of several major factors: (1) the increasing popularity of cocaine among the adult population, including its use by famous athletes, entertainers, business executives, and professionals who serve as role models for youngsters of all ages; (2) the perpetuation of cocaine's image as a chic, upper-class, nonaddictive, relatively harmless, intoxicant which produces a sensational "high"; (3) the abundance of cocaine supplies, and at reduced prices, which has made the drug more accessible; and (4) the appearance of "crack" on the illicit drug market which has provided adolescents with direct access to smokable cocaine freebase, a highly addictive form of cocaine, at a price almost any teenager can afford.[2]

2. PHARMACOLOGY

Cocaine hydrochloride powder is the most popular form of cocaine available in the United States. It is a white, crystalline substance typically sold on the illicit drug market in units of a gram, ranging in price from $75 to $100 per gram. Heavy users may purchase cocaine supplies in larger quantities and at reduced prices, either by the ounce (approximately 28 grams), "quarter" (approximately 7 grams), or "eighth" (approximately 3.5 grams).[3]

Cocaine hydrochloride powder is readily absorbed into the bloodstream via the nasal mucosa. Thus, nasal inhalation or "snorting" is an effective and popular route of cocaine administration. Because it is soluble in water, cocaine hydrochloride can be administered intravenously. When cocaine and heroin are mixed together in the same syringe, the drug combination is known as a "speedball."

Cocaine powder is not smokable because the active drug decomposes at the temperatures achieved by a match or lighter. However, using a simple chemical procedure, the powder can be readily transformed into a smokable form of the drug known as freebase or "crack."[4] The procedure can be performed quickly and cheaply using baking soda, heat, and water. Freebase and crack are synonymous. Crack is not a new drug, but a new way of packaging and selling freebase cocaine. Before the appearance of crack, anyone who wanted to smoke cocaine freebase had to buy cocaine powder and then perform the chemical conversion process themselves. The selling of crack on the illicit drug market makes the smokable cocaine freebase directly available to the consumer. Crack (and the way it is packaged) is especially attractive to adolescents for several reasons. Smoking generates an instantaneous and extremely intense euphoria or "rush." This stems directly from the highly rapid and efficient absorption of cocaine by the pulmonary route of administration. Crack is sold in very small dosage units of ready-to-smoke "rocks" that cost as little as $5 or $10 each, placing the drug within financial reach of almost any teenager. These rocks are dispensed in tiny plastic vials that are easily concealed and convenient to carry. Smoking cocaine is invariably perceived by potential users as less invasive, "sick," or dangerous than injecting it, although there are actually few differences between the results of these two methods of administration in terms of absorption, magnitude of drug effects, and addiction potential. Not only does smoking cocaine have a more benign connotation than injecting it, but many potential crack users already have experience and familiarity with other drugs (e.g., marijuana and nicotine), which further reduces the barriers to experimentation with crack.

Cocaine is a tropane alkaloid extracted from the leaves of the coca plant, Erythloxylon coca. Cocaine has three principal pharmacologic actions: it is a local anesthetic, a peripheral sympathomimetic, and a potent CNS stimulant.[3]

The psychoactive use of cocaine by humans stems from the drug's ability to chemically alter brain function and thereby induce feelings of stimulation and euphoria. Cocaine's effects on the CNS are complex and its mechanism of action is not well understood. When used intermittently, cocaine stimulates the release and inhibits the reuptake of dopamine and norepinephrine in selected areas of the brain. Chronic use leads to depletion of dopamine and other neurotransmitters. These neurochemical changes caused by chronic use may be the physiological substrate of compulsive cocaine use and addiction.[5]

3. HEALTH CONSEQUENCES

The mood-altering effects of cocaine are especially appealing to adolescents. Cocaine produces intense feelings of euphoria, energy, and confidence. In the early stages of cocaine involvement, users often feel more talkative, sociable, adventurous, and sexual. Cocaine can instantly overcome shyness, awkwardness, boredom, stress, sexual inhibitions, and low self-esteem. For many, it is the ultimate escape from negative mood states. Cocaine use is often referred to as "partying" by those who have come to expect good feelings and decreased inhibitions from cocaine. These are highly attractive benefits to many adolescents, particularly those who may look for any opportunity to celebrate and "let loose."

A pattern of escalating cocaine use and dependency is promoted to some extent by the drug's unique pharmacologic properties. The "high" is extremely pleasurable, but short-lived, leading to a pattern of repeated dosing at short intervals in order to maintain the desired mood state. As usage becomes regular and intensified, the brief euphoria is followed immediately by an unpleasant rebound dysphoria, or "crash," that leaves the user feeling uncomfortable and desiring an immediate return to the euphoric state. The crash from cocaine typically leads to the abuse of alcohol and other sedative-hypnotics, as the user attempts to alleviate the unpleasant feelings. As tolerance to cocaine develops, many users find themselves "chasing" the original high, which is vividly remembered.[6]

Both tolerance and dependence occur with chronic cocaine use. Decreased intensity or disappearance of the cocaine-induced euphoria usually occurs with repeated doses, particularly when there is a pattern of intensive use. Larger doses may temporarily override an existing tolerance to these effects, but at a certain point most intensive users become refractory to the cocaine-induced euphoria, irrespective of the amount of drug that is taken. Dependence on cocaine is evidenced by a loss of control over use, urges and cravings for the drug, and continued use despite adverse medical and psychosocial consequences. There is usually no dramatic physical withdrawal syndrome associated with abrupt cessation of chronic cocaine use. Nonetheless, cocaine is still considered to be physically addictive since it produces significant biochemical changes in brain activity that appear to give rise to cravings and urges that propel compulsive drug-taking behavior. The notion that cocaine is psychologically but not physically addictive is no longer considered valid by most drug experts. The greatest danger of cocaine by far is its high addiction potential. Even in reasonably stable, well-functioning adolescents, cocaine may acquire control of the user's behavior.[6]

Serious physiologic and somatic consequences tend to be uncommon in cocaine users, even in high-dose, chronic users. Death rates from cocaine use are low, despite publicity suggesting the contrary. However, potentially fatal toxic reactions to cocaine do occur; these include brain seizures, stroke, respiratory arrest, cardiac arrhythmias, and hypertension.[7] The most common types of medical problems stemming from cocaine use are usually related to the route of drug administration. Intranasal users may experience rhinorrhea, sinus headaches, nasal congestion, nasal sores, and nasal bleeding. Chronic freebase smokers may experience chest congestion, wheezing, and sore throat from inhaling the hot cocaine vapors. Intravenous users tend to experience the most serious drug-related medical problems, resulting mainly from their use of needles.[8] As with other intravenously abused drugs, these problems include abscesses at injection sites, hepatitis, endocarditis, and exposure to AIDS.

The most obvious and severe consequences of chronic cocaine use are behavioral, psychological, and social dysfunction. Unfortunately, cocaine use often is not evident until the problem has progressed to the point of serious abuse and dependency. Early warning signs are rarely present or recognized, except when the adolescent is actually found to be using or possessing cocaine. Common symptoms in regular or intensive users may include mood swings, irritability, short temper, depression, memory impairment, chronic lassitude, erratic sleep patterns (insomnia, excessive sleeping, or both), social withdrawal, and loss of interest in school, hobbies, sports, and family. More severe symptoms may include paranoia, suicidal ideation, and violence. As the user becomes increasingly obsessed with cocaine, all other aspects of functioning tend to deteriorate.[8] Cocaine abuse during pregnancy has been associated with an increased rate of spontaneous abortions and stillbirths related to abruptio placenta.[9] Although teratogenicity has been demonstrated in mice, the relationship of cocaine to congenital abnormalities in humans remains unclear.[10] Current evidence would suggest an increase in malformations, in particular bony skull defects. Babies born to addicted mothers have been noted to demonstrate depressed interactive behavior, difficulty with arousal, and irritability once aroused.[3] The relationship of these observations to subsequent neuropsychological problems remains unproven. An increased rate of unexplained sudden death during the first month of life has been suggested but remains unconfirmed. To date, no specific neonatal withdrawal syndrome requiring pharmacologic therapy has been described.

4. LABORATORY EVALUATION

Cocaine can be detected in urine and blood. However, because cocaine is rapidly metabolized, reliable detection of the drug requires sophisticated testing methodology such as enzyme-immunoassay or radioimmunoassay procedures which can yield accurate results for up to 48-72 hours after cocaine use.[3]

5. TREATMENT CONSIDERATIONS

Treatment of severe overdose reactions may require heroic measures, including respiratory assistance and a life-support system. Physiologic compromise is often complicated by the presence of other drugs. No specific pharmacologic antagonist to cocaine is available.[4]

Treatment of cocaine addiction is best conducted within the context of a highly structured chemical dependency treatment program.[11] The program should include: (1) immediate, total abstinence from cocaine and all other mood-altering substances; (2) individual, group, and family counseling; (3) supervised urine testing at least two to three times per week; and, (4) the application of specific relapse-prevention techniques. Most cocaine abusers do not require hospitalization, since there is no withdrawal syndrome that necessitates intensive medical management. However, inpatient treatment may be needed when there is (1) physical dependency on sedative-hypnotics or alcohol (2) suicidal, violent, or psychotic behavior and (3) inability to achieve abstinence despite outpatient treatment. There is no known effective pharmacotherapy for cocaine dependence. Experimental trials with a variety of agents, including antidepressants, lithium, bromocriptine, and others, have yielded inconsistent and unimpressive findings.[12] None of these trials has been conducted in adolescents. The most effective treatment programs combine professional interventions with self-help focusing on behavioral and attitudinal change, development of a drug-free lifestyle, and maintenance of long-term sobriety.

REFERENCES

1.   Johnston LD, O'Malley PM, Bachman JG: *Drug Use by High School Seniors - The Class of 1986*, US Department of Health and Human Services publication No. (ADM) 87-1535. Rockville, MD, 1987
2.   Cohen S: Causes of the cocaine outbreak, in Washton AM, Gold MS (eds): *Cocaine: A Clinician's Handbook*. New York, Guilford Press 1987; pp 3-9
3.   Mofenson HC, Caraccio TR: Cocaine. *Pediatr Ann* 1987;16:864-874
4.   Abramowicz M (ed): Adverse effects of cocaine abuse. *MedLett Drug Ther* 1984; 26:51-52
5.   Koob GT, Vaccarino FJ, Amalric M, et al: Neural substates for cocaine and opiate reinforcement, in Fisher S, Raskin A, and Uhlenhuth EM (eds): *Cocaine: Clinical and Behavioral Aspects*. New York, Oxford University Press, 1987, pp 80-108
6.   Jones RT: Psychopharmacology of cocaine, in Washton AM, and Gold MS (eds): *Cocaine: A Clinician's Handbook*. New York, Guilford Press, 1987, pp 55-72

7. Wetli CV, Wright RK: Death caused by recreational cocaine use. *JAMA* 1979; 241:2519-2522

8. Estroff TW: Medical and biological consequences of cocaine abuse, in Washton AM, and Gold MS (eds): *Cocaine: A Clinician's Handbook*. New York, Guilford Press, 1987, pp 23-32

9. Bingol N, Fuchs M, Diaz V, et al: Teratogenicity of cocaine in humans. *J Pediatr* 1987; 110:93-96

10. Mahalik MP, Gautier RF, Mann DE, et al: Teratogenic potential of cocaine hydrochloride in CF-1 mice. *J Pharm Sci* 1980; 69:703-709

11. Morehouse ER: Treating adolescent cocaine abuses, in Washton AM, and Gold MS (eds): *Cocaine: A Clinician's Handbook*. New York, Guilford Press, 1987, pp 135-151

12. Kleber HD, Gawin FH: Pharmacological treatments of cocaine abuse, in Washton AM, and Gold MS (eds): *Cocaine: A Clinician's Handbook*. New York, Guilford Press, 1987, pp 118-134

INHALANTS

1. EPIDEMIOLOGY

Inhaling volatile gases such as nitrous oxide or ether for their mind-altering effects was quite popular among adults in the nineteenth century. However, abuse of inhalants by adolescents became a concern in the United States in the early 1960s, with the epidemic of glue sniffing among children and young teenagers. Through the 1970s and 1980s, other volatile substances and aerosols came into widespread use as inhalants.

Epidemiologic surveys of inhalant use are somewhat difficult to interpret because the wording of the questions is inconsistent from survey to survey. Some ask only about glue sniffing, whereas others include questions about inhalation of gasoline, other solvents, aerosols, and nitrites. The annual national surveys of high school seniors between 1979 and 1986 reveal that 18%-20% of these young people consistently report inhalant use.[1] However, fewer than 3% of respondents reported using inhalants in the 30 days prior to the survey. Inhalant use appears to be more popular in the southwest, especially among Pueblo Indian and Mexican-American adolescents.[2] Much of the inhalant use among young adolescents is experimental and it often occurs as a group activity. Substances such as airplane glue, gasoline, spray paints, aerosols used as propellants for deodorants, cleaning fluids, Scotch-Guard®, and typewriter correction fluid (e.g., Liquid Paper®, White Out®), are legal, inexpensive, and readily available. School authorities and parents are not likely to become suspicious when they encounter a 13-year-old with a can of deodorant.

Gasoline sniffing has been reported as a recreational behavior since the early 1970s, especially among children in certain ethnic and sociocultural groups. Several reports from the United States, Canada, and Australia document a very high prevalence of gasoline sniffing among native Indian or aboriginal children living in isolated areas.[3] In addition, the prevalence of this behavior is high among economically disadvantaged young adolescents, particularly those in the southwestern United States.

The volatile nitrites such as amyl, butyl, or isobutyl nitrite became popular in the 1970s among male homosexuals as enhancers of the sexual experience. Epidemiologic data specific to the adolescent population are rare in the literature, although 5% of 1986 high school seniors reported using nitrites within the 12 months prior to the survey.[1] In one study, a survey of 173 13-22-year-olds in a long-term drug treatment facility, 43% admitted to having used isobutyl nitrite at least once and 13% had used it ten or more times.[4] A minority of these youths had used the drug in conjunction with a sexual experience; for those who did, it was heterosexual not homosexual intercourse.

2. PHARMACOLOGY

Inhalation is accomplished in a variety of ways. The volatile substance may be poured or sprayed into a plastic bag and inhaled from the bag. Liquid hydrocarbons such as solvents or cleaning fluids can be inhaled from soaked rags placed over the mouth and nose. Butyl or isobutyl nitrite are sold in small glass bottles in "head shops" and pornography stores or by mail order. Carrying street names such as "Rush," "Locker Room," "Bullet," "Quicksilver," and "Thrust." These drugs may be inhaled directly from the bottle. The prescription variety of amyl nitrite ("poppers"), used as a vasodilator in the treatment of angina pectoris, comes in a small glass vial that is crushed (popped) prior to inhalation.

The chemicals in most inhalants are rapidly absorbed in the lungs and exert their central nervous system effects within seconds, producing an altered mental state for about five to fifteen minutes. Tolerance often develops in chronic users, but withdrawal symptoms are rare.

3. HEALTH CONSEQUENCES

Toluene is the most common hydrocarbon found in paints, lacquer thinners, and household and model glues. Inhalation of this chemical as well as other hydrocarbons has been associated with renal and hepatic damage, peripheral neuropathy, convulsions, encephalopathy, and other CNS toxicity.[5] Sudden death associated with both glue-sniffing and especially with inhalation of aerosols containing halogenated hydrocarbons (Freons) has been reported in a number of adolescents.[6] These deaths are thought to be due to cardiac arrhythmias resulting from sensitization of the heart to epinephrine.[6] This mechanism is similar to that which is known to occur with halothane, a related chemical that is used as an anesthetic agent. The death is often reported to occur while the intoxicated teenager is running or very agitated due to hallucinations and presumably experiencing an increase in the secretion of epinephrine.

Gasoline sniffing has been associated with ataxia, chorea, tremor, organic lead encephalopathy, hepatic damage, peripheral neuropathy, and myopathy.[3] It is virtually certain that chronic gasoline abusers suffer neuropsychologic and intellectual deficits secondary to lead poisoning.

Trichloromethane, perchloroethylene, and trichloroethylene found in Scotch-Guard®, Carbona® spot remover, Liquid Paper® typewriter correction fluid, and some glues have been implicated in acute hepatic and renal toxicity and also in sudden death from cardiac arrhythmias.[7] King, et al., report the sudden deaths of four adolescents immediately after inhaling the vapors from typewriter correction fluid.[8] Toxicologic analysis revealed trichloromethane, trichloroethylene, or both, in blood samples from all four patients. None had ethanol detected in their blood. None showed evidence at autopsy of acute liver or kidney damage. The cause of all four deaths was thought to be cardiac arrhythmia.

Inhaling amyl, butyl, or isobutyl nitrite has been reported to cause headaches, tachycardia, syncope, and hypotension due to the vasodilator effects.[9] These substances have also been associated with increased intraocular pressure and with methemoglobinemia leading to cyanosis and hypoxia. People with glaucoma and with significant anemia who use nitrates are at particular risk; however, few deaths have been reported.

4. LABORATORY EVALUATION

Specific testing for most inhalants is difficult because of their rapid elimination and volatility. Because of the frequency of hepatic, renal, and hematologic damage caused by these substances, however, complete blood counts, coagulation studies, liver function tests, and renal function tests should be performed on all inhalant abusers. For gasoline sniffers, blood lead concentration should be determined since the blood lead level has been found to be elevated even in children who have only sniffed gasoline a few times.[3]

5. TREATMENT CONSIDERATIONS

Treatment should be similar to that offered to adolescents with other substance-abuse problems and should include, for those who are deeply involved, consideration of residential or community-based drug-treatment programs and family involvement. Chelation therapy is effective for tetraethyl lead toxicity from gasoline inhalation.

REFERENCES

1. Johnston LD, O'Malley PM, Bachman JG: *Drug Use by High School Seniors - The Class of 1986*, US Department of Health and Human Services publication No. (ADM) 87-1535. Rockville, MD, 1987
2. Werner M: Inhalant Abuse. *PharmChem Newsletter* 1979; 8:36-51
3. Fortenberry DJ: Gasoline sniffing. *Amer J Med* 1985; 79:740-744
4. Schwartz RH, Peary P: Abuse of isobutyl nitrite inhalation (Rush) by adolescents. *Clin Pediatr* 1986; 25(6):308-310
5. Anon.: Treatment of acute drug abuse reactions. *Med Lett Drugs Ther* 1987; 29(748):83-86
6. Bass M: Sudden sniffing death. *JAMA* 1970; 212(12): 2075-2079
7. Litt IF, Cohen MI: Danger...vapour harmful: spot remover sniffing. *N Engl J Med* 1969; 281:543-544
8. King GS, Smialek JE, Troutman WG: Sudden death in adolescents resulting from the inhalation of typewriter correction fluid. *JAMA* 1985; 253(11)1604-1606
9. Cohen S: The volatile nitrites. *JAMA* 1979; 241(19):2077-2078

STIMULANTS

1. EPIDEMIOLOGY

Amphetamines first achieved widespread use in the U.S. during the early 1950s, and they were prescribed until recently for common conditions such as obesity, mild depression, and fatigue. Now, however, they are considered to have a high potential for abuse and are Schedule II controlled drugs. The only uses for which they are considered effective and indicated are narcolepsy and hyperkinetic behavior in children. Concurrent with the introduction of amphetamines as therapeutic agents was a surge in their popularity as drugs of abuse. Such abuse has ranged from occasional self-medication for obesity or fatigue to prolonged amphetamine binges. Amphetamines as drugs of abuse are known by a multitude of street names including "speed," "black beauties," "BAM" (crushed tablets injected intravenously, sometimes with heroin), "mollies," "bennies," "splash," and "uppers." The proportion of high school seniors who had amphetamines prescribed for them dropped from 15% to 7% between 1976 and 1982; however, the rate has remained fairly constant since that time.[1] It is likely that this medically supervised use is at least partially responsible for the fact that after marijuana, amphetamines had the highest rates of current use (7%) among high school seniors in 1986. In that year, amphetamines had been used at least once by 23% of these students.[1]

Another group of drugs, the amphetamine "look alikes," have become problematic in recent years. These drugs, most of which contain phenylpropanolamine (PPA) or PPA and caffeine, are sold over the counter or through mailorder houses and are thus widely available. They are promoted as treatments for weight loss. When taken in large enough doses, they are capable of producing the "high" as well as the adverse side effects associated with the amphetamines.

2. PHARMACOLOGY

Amphetamine, the name of a specific chemical (alphamethylphenylethylamine) is the parent compound for the class of stimulants known as amphetamines, including DL-amphetamine (Benzedrine®), dextroamphetamine (Dexedrine®), and methamphetamine. A number of amphetamine analogues also exist; these include benzphetamine hydrochloride, chlorphentermine hydrochloride, fenfluramine hydrochloride, phendimetrazine tartrate, and many others. All have properties very similar to those of the amphetamines. The amphetamine "look alikes" mentioned above are actually sympathomimetic agents whose chemical structure is quite different from that of the amphetamine analogues.

Although the mechanism of action of the amphetamines is not entirely understood, it is clear that the norepinephrine- and dopamine-mediated systems of the brain are involved. The amphetamines may exert their effects either by preventing catecholamine reuptake or by facilitating release of catecholamines from the presynaptic neuron. An alternative explanation is that they directly affect catecholamine receptors by inhibiting monoamine oxidase.[2] In any case, clinical manifestations are produced from a direct effect on adrenergic receptors in muscles and glands as well as from stimulation of the medullary respiratory center and the cerebrospinal axis.

The amphetamines are well absorbed from the gastrointestinal tract, after which they undergo deamination and hydroxylation in the liver. Accumulated hydroxylated metabolites have been implicated in the development of the psychosis sometimes associated with amphetamine use. Finally, the unchanged amphetamines and the metabolized forms are excreted through the kidneys. They can be detected in the urine between three hours and three days after ingestion.

3. HEALTH CONSEQUENCES

Within approximately 30 minutes of oral ingestion or five minutes following subcutaneous injection amphetamines begin to exert their effects. Effects begin almost instantly after intravenous administration, and they are extremely intense.

Amphetamine use results in an initial "rush" or feeling of extreme exhilaration, that is followed by a more sustained period of euphoria, greater ability to concentrate, wakefulness, depressed appetite, self-confidence, and excitement. Pre-existing fatigue or depression are immediately abolished. Tolerance quickly develops, and chronic users develop confusion, paranoia, headache, and depression. Many chronic users will have a history of weight loss, and may seem to be agitated or paranoid. Dilated pupils, hypertension, and tachycardia, are among the more frequent physical findings.[2]

Manifestations of mild amphetamine toxicity include restlessness, irritability, insomnia, tremor, hyper-reflexia, diaphoresis, dilated pupils, and flushing. With increasing dosage the adolescent will experience confusion, hypertension, tachypnea, and mild temperature elevation. With more severe toxicity, delirium, hypertensive crisis, dysrhythmias, seizures, coma, cardiovascular collapse, and death may occur.[2] PPA, the "look alike amphetamine," has been reported to cause hypertension, psychosis, and cerebral hemorrhage, although some controversy exists as to the extent of the effect. As with other drugs, intravenous use of amphetamines may be associated with pulmonary granulomata or emboli due to the injection of talc or starch, as well as with hepatitis and other infectious complications resulting from sharing unsterile needles.

Tolerance and physical dependence occur with regular heavy use of amphetamines, and an abstinence syndrome will occur upon cessation of their use. Depression is the most prominent manifestation of stimulant drug withdrawal. It reaches its peak two to three days after the last dose is taken. The mood swing may be so severe that it is accompanied by suicidal or homicidal ideation. Exhaustion, prolonged sleep, and voracious appetite also occur; however, severe reactions such as seizures or death have not been reported.[2]

Amphetamine psychosis, which usually occurs in chronic users, has also been reported to occur after a single large dose. This drug-induced psychosis may be confused with schizophrenia. The hallucinations that occur with use of these drugs are most often visual, tactile, or olfactory, as compared with the auditory hallucinations associated with paranoid schizophrenia. Repetitive, stereotyped, compulsive behaviors that are probably dopamine related are also observed in chronic users. Symptoms of psychosis begin to fade within a few days after cessation of drug use. The amphetamine analogues have also been associated with a drug-induced psychosis.

Limb deformities, biliary atresia, and other birth defects have occurred in babies born to mothers who have used amphetamines during the first trimester of pregnancy.[4,5] Furthermore, a neonatal withdrawal syndrome consisting of diaphoresis, irritability, hypoglycemia, tremulousness, and even seizures has been reported.[6]

4. **LABORATORY EVALUATION**

Urine and blood assays for amphetamines are widely available and will remain positive for two days after the last dose (See Chapter 4).

5. **TREATMENT CONSIDERATIONS**

Manifestations of amphetamine overdose are often severe and life-threatening. If the drug has been taken orally, and the patient is awake, ipecac syrup, followed by activated charcoal and a cathartic such as magnesium citrate, should be administered.[2] A quiet environment with minimal external stimuli should be provided while hyperthermia and hypertension are treated. The central nervous system stimulant effects may be treated with chlorpromazine or droperidol. Chlorpromazine should be used only when the diagnosis of amphetamine toxicity is certain, as it is contraindicated in the treatment of the psychosis induced by phencyclidine and the hallucinogens. Treatment of the abstinence syndrome from stimulants includes several days of professional support and protective supervision within a hospital environment. Pharmacologic detoxification is unnecessary.

REFERENCES

1. Johnston JD, O'Malley PM, Bachman JG: *Drug Use by High School Seniors - The Class of 1986*, US Department of Health and Human Services publication No. (ADM) 87-1535. Rockville, MD, 1987
2. Litovitz T: Amphetamines, in Haddad LM, Winchester JF (eds):*Clinical Management of Poisoning and Drug Overdose*, Philadelphia, WB Saunders, 1983, pp 469-475
3. Kulberg A: Substance abuse: Clinical identification and management. *Pediatr Clin North Am* 1986; 33:325-361
4. Nelson MM, Forfar JO: Associations between drugs administered during pregnancy and congenital abnormalities of the fetus. *Br Med J* 1971; 523-527

5. Levin JN: Amphetamine ingestion with biliary atresia. *JPediatr* 1971; 79:130-131
6. Larsson G: The amphetamine addicted mother and her child. *Acta Paediatr Scand* 1980; 278(suppl):1-24

HALLUCINOGENS

1. EPIDEMIOLOGY

Naturally occurring hallucinogenic substances have been used in certain cultures for thousands of years, mainly in religious ceremonies. Members of the native American church use peyote, a cactus plant containing mescaline, believing that it enables them to commune more easily with God. In a similar fashion, native populations of Mexico use mushrooms containing the hallucinogen psilocybin in their religious rites. Lysergic acid diethylamide (LSD) is the potent hallucinogenic drug that became popular in the United States during the "psychedelic era" of the 1960s. LSD does not occur naturally and was first synthesized in 1938 at Sandoz Laboratories in Switzerland.[1]

When hallucinogenic substances first came into widespread use in the mid-1960s, a small but significant number of young people used them on a daily or almost daily basis. Today, however, these drugs are largely used on an experimental basis—once, or at most a few times, a year. The prevalence of adolescents who have ever used a hallucinogen also appears to be decreasing. In 1979, 18.6% of high school seniors had tried a hallucinogenic substance; by 1986, this had decreased to 12% and only about half of these students had used a hallucinogen within the past year.[2]

2. PHARMACOLOGY

The hallucinogens probably exert their effects by modifying neurotransmitter pathways in the brain. The chemical structure of the neurotransmitter serotonin involves an indole nucleus, and both LSD and psilocybin contain an indole ring in their chemical structures.[1] Mescaline contains a catechol nucleus similar to that found in the catecholamine-type neurotransmitters such as noradrenaline. DOM 2,5-dimethoxy-4-methylamphetamine (STP) is a synthetic catechol-type hallucinogen. Other hallucinogens act on the neurotransmitter acetylcholine. A number of plants such as the deadly nightshade (belladonna) contain cholinergic hallucinogens. Jimson ("Loco") weed contains atropine and scopolamine, potent acetylcholine blockers, and is used by some adolescents for its mind-altering properties.

LSD is the most potent of the hallucinogens. It is effective orally in minute doses (in the order of 30-50 micrograms per dose).[1] Mescaline is 4,000 times less potent and psilocybin is approximately 100-200 times less potent than LSD.[3] Most of these indole- and catechol-type hallucinogens are sold as tablets or powders. However, LSD, which is easily dissolved, is often sold absorbed onto a piece of blotting paper ("blotter acid") and is ingested paper and all. Psilocybin can also be ingested in the form of "magic mushrooms" that have been gathered in the wild or cultivated indoors.[4] Drug effects begin 40-60 minutes after ingestion and peak approximately three or four hours after being taken. Effects of the drug may last up to 8-12 hours. The most striking effect of LSD and similar hallucinogens is a dramatic alteration in visual perception.[1] Colors seem brighter and are often split into the full spectrum so that objects appear to have rainbows around them. The shape and size of objects are distorted, and their boundaries seem to shift and dissolve. Synesthesia, a mixing of senses, is common, and users often say that they can visualize music as a series of colors and shapes. Most users realize that these perceptual changes are caused by the drug and can remember them when the "trip" is over.[1] Thus, they are not true hallucinations but "pseudo-hallucinations" or illusions. Very high doses of these drugs, however, can produce frank visual hallucinations. Accompanying these visual perceptual distortions are mood changes, feelings of depersonalization, and some, usually minimal, somatic symptoms such as tremors, dizziness, nausea, and tingling. The emotional reactions to the drug experience can vary from panic to a transcendental feeling of union with the universe.[1] Tolerance appears to develop with frequent use of any of the indole- or catechol-type hallucinogens but this tolerance is short-lived, disappearing after a week or two of abstinence.

The anticholinergic-type of hallucinogens such as Jimson weed, produce a different syndrome of intoxication with many more physiological disturbances due to their peripheral as well as central effects.[5] Users experience true visual hallucinations and have no concurrent awareness that they are drug-induced. Because of this, panic, combative behavior, and disorientation are much more common than with LSD. In addition, signs of peripheral anticholinergic effects are prominent; these include mydriasis, flushed faces, dry mucous membranes, tachycardia, and, in some cases, fever, hypertension, urinary retention, and convulsions.[5]

3. HEALTH CONSEQUENCES

The toxicity of the indole- and catechol-type hallucinogens appears to be mainly psychological. Used under controlled conditions such as religious ceremonies or laboratory experiments, they appear to be quite safe from a physiologic standpoint. However, it is essential to remember that the purity of "street drugs" is always in question. The naturally occurring hallucinogens such as mescaline are very expensive, and on the illicit drug market, misrepresenting such substances with the less costly and more potent LSD or PCP is the norm.

The adverse psychological effects of the hallucinogens occur in three areas. Panic attacks during the height of the drug experience (a "bad trip") are common.[1] Individuals can become quite distraught and are at risk for accidents unless they are supervised and protected by lay or medical caretakers. Psychotic reactions may be precipitated by the drug experience, often in people with significant psychiatric difficulties prior to the drug ingestion.[1] These psychoses often require long-term treatment. There have been occasional reports of suicides during drug-induced psychosis. A disturbing effect that has been reported with hallucinogens is the "flashback," an unwanted repetition of the drug experience without the ingestion of drugs. Flashbacks seem to occur during times of psychological stress and diminish in frequency and intensity the longer the individual refrains from use of hallucinogenic drugs.[1]

LSD has not been shown to be a teratogen in humans despite the "chromosome breakage" publicity of the late 1960s. Nonetheless, it is prudent to recommend abstinence from any recreational drug during pregnancy.

The anticholinergic hallucinogens appear to have more potential for physiologic harm for several reasons: (1) effects may last for days rather than hours; (2) the intoxicated person is disoriented, cannot be reasoned with and must usually be physically restrained; and (3) large overdoses can cause convulsions, severe hypertension, or coma with respiratory depression.[5]

4. TREATMENT CONSIDERATIONS

Acute intoxication with LSD or other indole- or catechol-type hallucinogens should be treated by removing the individual to a quiet, nonthreatening environment and "talking him down," that is, repeatedly reassuring him or her that these experiences are drug-related and that they will eventually disappear.[1] Agitation and panic can be treated with a benzodiazepine or haloperidol. Flashbacks often require only reassurance or a mild tranquilizer. The adolescent with flashbacks should be cautioned to avoid not only hallucinogens but also marijuana and antihistamines, which can trigger these experiences. Prolonged psychotic reactions require psychiatric intervention.

Treatment of anticholinergic-type hallucinogen intoxication requires hospitalization because of the long-lasting mental effects of these drugs.[5] Gastric lavage is indicated in all cases, even if the ingestion occurred hours or days prior to medical treatment because of the markedly decreased gastric motility associated with atropine poisoning. Intravenous fluids and urinary catheterization may be required. Sedation can be achieved with benzodiazepines or barbiturates. Phenothiazines should be avoided because of their additive anticholinergic effects. Physostigmine is of questionable efficacy and, when used at all, should be reserved for life-threatening overdoses.[5]

REFERENCES

1. Ray O: *Drugs, Society and Human Behavior.* 3rd edition, St.Louis, C.V. Mosby Co., 1983, pp 373-397
2. Johnston LD, O'Malley PM, Bachman JG: *Drug Use by High School Seniors - The Class of 1986,* US Department of Health and Human Services publication No. (ADM) 87-1535. Rockville, MD, 1987
3. Anon.: Mescaline. *PharmChem Newsletter* 1(4):1972
4. Beck JE, Gordon DV: Psilocybian Mushrooms. *PharmChem Newsletter* 1982, 4(1):1-4
5. Shervette RE, Schydlower M, Lampe RM, et al: Jimson "loco"weed abuse in adolescents. *Pediatrics* 1979; 63(4):520-523

PHENCYCLIDINE (PCP)

1. EPIDEMIOLOGY

It is difficult to quantify the use of this illicit, hallucinogenic substance since many users themselves do not know that they have taken it. On the street, PCP is often sold as mescaline, THC, or psilocybin, and it is frequently used as an adulterant in other illicit products. The latest National Institute on Drug Abuse (NIDA) survey of substance abuse among teenagers indicates that 12% of high school seniors in 1986 reported hallucinogen use and that many of the hallucinogens probably contained PCP.[1] Three percent of 1985 seniors reported knowingly using PCP within the last year. In a recent study among 202 general adolescent clinic patients at an urban children's hospital, 18 patients were found to have a positive urine test for PCP.[2] All of these adolescents also had cannabinoid metabolites in their urine. None of the 128 patients without cannabinoid metabolites in their urine had a positive urine screen for PCP. The concordance between a self-reported history of use and confirmatory urine test was higher for marijuana use than for PCP, 91% vs 11% suggesting to the authors the possibility that the adolescents were smoking PCP without knowing it.[2]

Phencyclidine was first used illicitly in 1967 in the Haight-Ashbury district of San Francisco, where it was sold as the "Peace Pill." It soon developed a bad reputation because of its propensity to cause "bad trips," and use declined. In the mid-1970s, new marketing strategies such as dusting the substance onto a leaf mixture for smoking, and misrepresenting PCP as some other less available substances, led to greatly increased use, especially in large cities. By the early 1980s, PCP was being described as the most frequently used hallucinogen in the United States. Most of the users are between 15 and 25 years of age. Phencyclidine is sold on the street as PCP, "Angel Dust," "Crystal," "Elephant (Monkey) Tranquilizer," "Hog," "Super Grass," "Angel Mist," "Peace Weed," and many other "brand" names. In addition, users often purchase PCP under the assumption that they are obtaining mescaline or another hallucinogen.

2. CLINICAL PHARMACOLOGY

Phencyclidine hydrochloride (l-[phenycyclohexyl] piperdine hydrochloride) was developed in the late 1950s by Parke Davis as an anesthetic agent with the brand name Sernyl®.[3] It initially seemed promising because it produced analgesia and sleep without causing respiratory or cardiovascular depression. A related drug, often used in pediatric anesthesia, is Ketamine®. The psychotoxic effects of PCP, however, made it unsuitable for use in humans, and for a while it was used legitimately only in veterinary medicine as a primate anesthetic called Sernylan®. This drug was taken off the market in the late 1970s and all the PCP now available is illegally manufactured. It is easily and inexpensively made by anyone with a rudimentary knowledge of organic chemistry. PCP is available as a white, crystalline powder that is readily soluble in water or alcohol. It can be dissolved and injected intravenously; snorted intranasally; ingested in food, beverages or as pills; or, most commonly, sprinkled (dusted) in powdered form over dried parsley, oregano, or marijuana leaves and smoked.

The route of administration determines the timing of onset of drug effects. Effects are felt within seconds of an intravenous dose, within two to five minutes after smoking or snorting the drug, and within 30 minutes of ingesting it. Maximum effect of the drug usually occurs 15 to 30 minutes after smoking or two to five hours after ingestion. The effects of PCP can last 12 hours or more, and drug-induced psychosis can last up to a month.

PCP is a weak base with a dissociation constant (pKa) of 8.5 and it is rapidly absorbed in the alkaline environment of the small bowel.[4] Most of the drug is rapidly metabolized to apparently inactive substances and excreted in the urine. More than 50% of an ingested dose is excreted in the urine as hydroxy and glucuronidyl metabolites within 12 hours. If the urine is acidified from pH7 to pH5, the PCP clearance rate increases one hundredfold.[4]

3. HEALTH CONSEQUENCES

In low doses (1-5 mg), PCP produces a feeling of euphoria and disinhibition with emotional lability much like drunkenness.[3,4,5] Moderate doses (5-10 mg) lead to a body-wide anesthetic effect with supersensitivity to sensations and impaired perceptions often resulting in panic reactions. Large doses (more than 10 mg) can produce a toxic psychosis indistinguishable from schizophrenia, with paranoia and auditory hallucinations and either excitement or stupor.[5] Massive overdoses can result in coma, seizures, rhabdomyolysis and, very rarely, apnea. Smoking or snorting the drug produces rapid effects and allows the user to control the dose better, thus decreasing the chance of toxic complications. Toxic reactions requiring medical attention more commonly follow ingestion rather than inhalation of PCP.[6] However, both passive (i.e., infants and children of abusers) and active smokers of the drug occasionally require treatment for acute short-term psychosis and also may require medical attention for accidents that have occurred during an altered state of consciousness.[6,7] It should be remembered that PCP is a potent analgesic; even if severely wounded, intoxicated individuals feel no pain.

The major effects of PCP, other than its effect on the mind, are sympathomimetic (tachycardia, hypertension, and hyperreflexia); cholinergic (constriction of the pupils [miosis], flushing, and increased sweating); and cerebellar (vertical and horizontal nystagmus, dysarthria, and ataxia).[3,4] Mental status can vary widely, from an excited, delirious, violent state to an unresponsive, calm, blankly staring state, to coma. The intoxicated individual experiences altered stereognosis and proprioception, numbness and analgesia, auditory or visual hallucinations, dysphoria, paranoia, and disorientation.[3,4] Very high doses of PCP have been associated with coma, cardiac arrhythmias, muscle rigidity, decerebrate or opisthotonic posturing, and rhabdomyolysis, leading to acute renal failure, seizures and death.[4,8]

Phencyclidine crosses the placenta and has been detected in the urine of newborn infants whose mothers had taken the drug up to three weeks prior to delivery.[9] Neonatal symptoms are similar to those occurring in mothers who have used opiates and include jitteriness, hypertonicity, and vomiting. Teratogenicity of the drug has been suggested but not proved. Accidental intoxication in infants and young children has been reported with increasing frequency since the late 1970s.[10] Hypertension and hyperflexia are uncommon in children under five years of age. The most frequent symptoms of PCP intoxication in young

children are lethargy, nystagmus, and opisthotonos.[10]
These nonspecific symptoms often resemble those of
meningitis, brain tumor, seizure disorder, and other types
of drug ingestion; thus, PCP should be specifically requested in the urine toxicology screening.

4. LABORATORY EVALUATION

The best method of screening for PCP intoxication is a
urine assay. One such assay, the enzyme-multiple immunoassay technique (EMIT) has a lower limit of sensitivity of 75 ng of PCP/mL of urine. Urine can also be
assayed for PCP by gas-liquid chromatography. The concentration of PCP in the urine bears little relation to the
degree of impairment in the user, however, since the
rapidity of excretion of the drug is variable and depends
on the pH of the urine. Blood concentration of PCP correlates more closely with symptoms and degree of toxicity,
but it is usually more difficult to obtain. (See Chapter 4).

5. TREATMENT CONSIDERATIONS

Acute transient toxic psychosis caused by smoking or
snorting PCP should be treated by protecting the individual from harm and minimizing the environmental
stimuli.[3,5] The patient should be placed in a dimly lit, quiet
room. "Talking down" should be avoided. Benzodiazepines,
such as Valium®, may be given for agitation: however,
other antipsychotic drugs should be avoided as they may
add to complications and have no proven effectiveness. If
the patient has ingested PCP, induction of emesis or gastric lavage is indicated since the drug is poorly absorbed
from the acidic stomach. Acidification of the urine with
either ascorbic acid or ammonium chloride will promote
more rapid excretion of the phencyclidine and may be helpful in shortening the duration of symptoms.[11] However,
large doses of either drug are required and, except when
there is physiologic compromise, there is seldom an ur-
gency to the alleviation of behavioral symptoms. This latter therapy should not be attempted in neonates because

of the dangers of a metabolic acidosis. Newborns are best treated with phenobarbital and observation.

REFERENCES

1. Johnston LD, O'Malley PM, Bachman JG: *Drug Use by High School Seniors - The Class of 1986*, US Department of Health and Human Services publication No. (ADM) 87-1535. Rockville, MD, 1987
2. Silber TJ, Josefson M, Hicks JM, et al: Prevalence of PCP use among adolescent marijuana users. *J Pediatr* 1988;112(5):872-879
3. Ray O: *Drugs, Society and Human Behavior*. 3rd edition, St.Louis, C.V. Mosby Co., 1983, pp 413-416
4. Goldfrank L, Osborn H: Phencyclidine (Angel Dust). *Hosp Physician* 1978; 5:18-21
5. Richards ML, Perry PJ, Liskow BI: Phencyclidine psychosis. *Drug Intell Clin Pharm* 1979; 13:336-339
6. Yesavage JA, Freman III AM: Acute phencyclidine (PCP) intoxication: psychopathology and prognosis. *J Clin Psychiatry* 1978; 39(8):664-666
7. Grove FE Jr.: Painless self-injury after ingestion of 'angel dust'. *JAMA* 1979; 242(7)655
8. Cogen FC, Rigg G, Simmons JL, et al: Phencyclidine associated acute rhabdomyolysis. *Ann Intern Med* 1978; 88:210-212
9. Strauss AA, Mondanlou HD, Bosu SK: Neonatal manifestations of maternal phencyclidine (PCP) abuse. *Pediatrics* 1981;68(4):550-552
10. Welch MJ, Correa GA: PCP intoxication in young children and infants. *Clin Pediatr* 1980; 19(8)510-514
11. Arnow R, Done AK: Phencyclidine overdose: an emerging concept of management. *JACEP* 1978; 7:56-59

OPIATES

1. EPIDEMIOLOGY

Opiates, particularly heroin and methadone, were major drugs of abuse among young people during the 1960s and early 1970s. While there has been a dramatic decline in the use of opiates since that time, a minority of young people continue to abuse them, and there has been a small but significant rise in use in recent years. Although 10% of high school seniors in 1986 reported some lifetime experience with opiates, daily use by these students was far less than 1%.[1] It should be noted, however, that opiate abuse and addiction are associated with dropping out of school and hence these teenagers would not be detected by an in-school survey. Furthermore, any incidence of intravenous drug abuse has become a matter of great concern in view of the relationship between such activity and acquired immunodeficiency syndrome (AIDS).

2. PHARMACOLOGY

The class of drugs called opiates includes morphine and codeine, which are actually derived from opium; heroin, oxycodone (in Percodan®, Percocet®, and Tylox®), and hydromorphone (Dilaudid®) which are semisynthetic; and methadone (Dolophine®), meperidine (Demerol®), propoxyphene (Darvon®, Darvocet®), and pentazocine (Talwin®), agents that are altogether synthetic. All of these drugs have an affinity to bind with stereospecific receptors in the brain. The range and intensity of the pharmacologic effects of each drug are largely dependent upon the relative binding affinity to the major central nervous system (CNS) receptors called mu, kappa, and sigma.[2] Taken orally, the opiates are readily absorbed from the gastrointestinal tract; however, first-pass extraction and metabolism by the microsomes in the endoplasmic reticulum of the liver result in less intense effects as compared with administration via the parenteral route.[3]

Heroin is a white, bitter, crystalline powder. When obtained by the user, it is usually mixed with lactose, which serves as a filler to dilute the opiate. Other substances such as quinine, procaine, or methylpyrilene are added to disguise the sweet taste of the lactose. The final concentration of heroin available to users varies from 1% to 20%, and a single dose may contain 1 to 20 mg of heroin.[4]

Instillation via the intranasal route, or "snorting," results in onset of psychopharmocologic effects in approximately 30 minutes. Snorting produces inflammation and erythema of the nasal mucosa, which preclude it from being used more frequently than every six hours or so. "Skin popping," or subcutaneous abuse, accelerates the onset of heroin's effects to 15 minutes. Intravenous abuse ("shooting up" or "mainlining") produces a very intense effect almost immediately.

Heroin is metabolized through hydrolyzation to 6-monoacetyl morphine and then to morphine, which is conjugated with glucuronic acid within the liver. It is excreted in the urine as free and conjugated morphine. Detoxification occurs rapidly; 90% of heroin is cleared from the body within 24 hours after administration. In the heroin addict, symptoms of an abstinence syndrome begin to occur approximately six hours after the last dose. In contrast, the effects of methadone, which is usually taken orally, begin within 30 minutes, and peak blood levels are reached in four to six hours. It is excreted quite slowly and has a plasma half-life of approximately 22 hours. The abstinence syndrome does not occur until more than 24 hours after the last dose.

3. HEALTH CONSEQUENCES

Although the major indication for the therapeutic use of the opiates is analgesia, the high potential for abuse of these drugs is related to their capacity to produce euphoria. Both of these effects are a result of activity in the opiate receptor sites of the brain. In addition to a direct analgesic effect, which is mediated via these receptors, the opiates produce an altered psychologic response to pain, suppression of anxiety, and sedation, all of which contribute to pain relief.

The somatic consequences of opiate abuse are related not only to the pharmacologic action of the drug but also, and even more frequently, to the method of drug administration and the lifestyle of the abuser. The lack of aseptic technique, the sharing of needles and syringes, and the presence of infectious agents that are admixed with the opiates results in a number of common, and often quite serious infectious complications. Cellulitis, skin abscesses, thrombophlebitis, endocarditis, intracranial and pulmonary abscesses, pneumonia, and hepatitis are among the infectious complications commonly encountered. Most recently, AIDS has become the infectious complication of intravenous abuse causing the greatest concern. Nearly 15,000 intravenous drug abusers in the United States have already been diagnosed as having AIDS, and that number is certain to rise.[5]

Among the consequences to the CNS secondary to opiate abuse is respiratory depression, a result of suppression of the medullary response to carbon dioxide, that causes a fall in the respiratory rate, minute volume, and tidal exchange. With overdose, there is the potential for respiratory arrest. The cough center, also located within the medulla, is similarly depressed, explaining the therapeutic use of opiates as antitussives but representing an additional danger with overdose. Other possible reactions to an overdose include pulmonary edema, an almost invariable feature; hypotension, with the potential for circulatory collapse which occurs secondary to vasodilation; and cardiopulmonary arrest.[3]

Beyond those CNS consequences associated with an overdose is the potential for cerebral abscesses. Such abscesses, which are often multiple and microscopic, may result from the direct injection of bacteria into the circulation or they may be secondary to septic embolization in the patient with endocarditis.[4] Peripheral neural complications include transverse myelitis and brachial and lumbosacral plexitis, which have been reported when individuals are re-exposed to heroin after a period of abstinence. These complications are rare in adolescents. A more common complication in adolescents is local anesthesia or ankle or wrist drop caused by accidental injection into, or adjacent to, a peripheral nerve.

Possible cardiopulmonary consequences of opiate abuse include orthostatic hypotension and syncope secondary to vasodilation. These cardiovascular effects usually do not occur with therapeutic doses of opiates or with amounts typically abused; however, as noted above, an acute opiate overdose may result in circulatory collapse and cardiopulmonary arrest. A frequent cardiac consequence is infective endocarditis. This may affect either the right or left side of the heart, the former being more common. Although bacteria, particularly *Staphylococcus aureus,* are most often the cause of this infection, fungal infections also occur and have a less favorable prognosis.[6] Septic embolization to the brain, spleen, kidneys, lungs, and bone has been observed with some frequency in patients with drug-related endocarditis. Pulmonary infections and edema, as noted above, are both rather constant components of an acute overdose reaction; other pulmonary consequences of intravenous opiate abuse are pulmonary hypertension and granulomata within the lung parenchyma. These are secondary to the deposition within the small blood vessels and tissue of the lung of inert fillers and impurities that have been mixed with heroin and enter the circulation at the time of injection.

Among the gastrointestinal effects of opiate abuse is a delay in gastric emptying time due to increased tone of the antral portion of the stomach and the proximal duodenum. Although this is accompanied by decreased production of hydrochloric acid and biliary and pancreatic secretions, the net effect favors duodenal ulcer formation.[7] Constipation is very common, due to a decrease in the propulsive contractions of the small and large intestine and increased ileocecal valve and anal sphincter tone. Tolerance does not develop to these gastrointestinal effects. The most frequent serious gastrointestinal complication of opiate abuse is viral hepatitis. The majority of intravenous abusers will eventually suffer a bout of viral hepatitis. Although in some cases this episode will be subclinical, a minority of patients will experience a fulminant course with hepatic decompensation, coma, and possibly death. More commonly, opiate abusers develop a chronic persistent hepatitis, with minimal elevations of hepatic enzymes and histologic evidence of periportal fibrosis.[8] This condition does not appear to require treatment; however, management would include periodic assessment of liver function.

Although opiates actually decrease libido, increased rates of sexually transmitted diseases are seen in drug-abusing adolescents most probably because of a lifestyle that often includes prostitution or promiscuity. It should be kept in mind that a reactive serologic test for syphilis (e.g., Venereal Disease Research Laboratory Test (VDRL)) may be due either to true infection or to a biologic false-positive test, which occurs frequently among heroin users.[9] The female opiate user may frequently experience amenorrhea and anovulatory cycles, and these young women experience a low rate of pregnancy despite their sexual activity. The disturbance of menstruation and ovulation probably occurs as a result of the effect of heroin on prolactin secretion.[10,11] The rate at which menses and ovulation resume after drug use is terminated varies inversely with the length of time that the opiate had been used. With abstinence, these adolescents will regain fertility and require contraception to avoid unwanted pregnancy.

The emergence of addiction to opiates is a function of the amount of drug abused and of the frequency and duration of that abuse. Although no exact formula can be defined for the development of addiction, it is clear that even the therapeutic use of daily opiates over a period of weeks may result in an abstinence syndrome upon withdrawal of the drug. Heroin and methadone result in the same symptomatology upon withdrawal; however, with methadone the onset does not occur until 24 to 48 hours after the last dose, while with heroin, symptoms usually occur within the first day. The opiate abstinence syndrome begins with yawning, restlessness, increased lacrimation, insomnia, and rhinorrhea, then progresses to mydriasis, piloerection (goose flesh), diaphoresis, flushing, tachycardia, hypertension, tremors and twitching, and later, muscle cramps, fever, nausea, vomiting, and intestinal hyperactivity with diarrhea. Seizures, one of the most severe manifestations of withdrawal, are quite rare in adolescents.[4] Women who have abused opiates during their pregnancies experience relatively higher rates of spontaneous abortions and stillbirths, and their infants are very often born small for gestational age. Maternal drug withdrawal during pregnancy, particularly during the third trimester, may increase the risk for fetal demise. A well-described abstinence syndrome, beginning from several hours to six weeks after delivery, occurs in newborns born to addicted mothers.[12] The time of onset and severity of the symptoms depend on the specific drug used (methadone withdrawal occurring later than heroin), the total daily dose used, duration of addiction, and the time of the last maternal dose. Symptoms range from mild irritability and feeding difficulty to seizures.

4. LABORATORY EVALUATION
Urine testing for the presence of opiates is widely available in most medical centers. Both thin-layer chromatography and radioimmunoassay techniques will detect opiate metabolites for several days after a last use (See Chapter 4).

5. TREATMENT CONSIDERATIONS
As noted previously, acute opiate overdose may result in respiratory depression, pulmonary edema, and cardiopulmonary arrest. Resuscitory efforts would include intubation and the administration of oxygen with positive end-expiratory pressure. The acute toxic effects of an opiate may be antagonized by the administration of naloxone, beginning with intermittent doses of 0.4 - 2.0 mg intravenously given as often as every two to three minutes. Bolus doses as high as 8 mg may be required. A continuous infusion with the administration of two thirds of the total initial dose each hour may be necessary, especially in cases of methadone intoxication in which the period of toxicity may be prolonged.[3] In addition, naloxone therapy may

be required for as long as a full day. As the duration of action of naloxone is much shorter than that of methadone, therapy should not be discontinued as soon as the patient regains consciousness. Relapse into coma may occur if naloxone therapy is discontinued prematurely. A radiograph of the chest should be performed to look for pneumonia or pulmonary edema. Antibiotics are given when either of these is present, as secondary infection commonly occurs with the latter.

Many adolescents will briefly experiment with heroin or methadone and not go on to addiction; nonetheless, these drugs must be considered highly addictive, and addiction to opiates carries a poor long-term prognosis. Adolescents who become addicted face a prolonged and even lifetime battle to achieve abstinence in which detoxification is but the first step. Treatment of the abstinence syndrome is aimed at maintaining patient comfort and preventing the rare but severe effects such as seizures. Detoxification should be viewed as preparation for entrance into a dependency treatment program. Few patients will continue to abstain from opiate use after detoxification without the benefit of therapeutic support. A variety of detoxification methods have been employed, including acupuncture, pharmacologic withdrawal, and abrupt cessation of drug use with behavioral support. Currently the most frequent method of detoxification involves the administration of methadone in a single daily dose of 30 to 40 mg, with that dose being reduced in 5 mg aliquots over time. By this method, abstinence can be attained in seven to ten days.[4] An alternate method is the administration of diazepam (Valium®) in a dose of 10 to 15 mg every four to six hours for three or four days.[4] Although this method has the advantages of avoiding the use of a substitute narcotic and more rapid detoxification, it is less likely to ablate all symptoms of withdrawal and hence is less well tolerated by adolescent addicts.

The long-term treatment of opiate addiction has primarily involved two modalities; drug-free therapeutic communities and methadone maintenance treatment pro-grams. Drug-free therapeutic communities vary in their approaches but most often share common themes of total drug abstinence, behavior modification, and self-help directed by ex-addicts rather than by behavioral pro-fessionals. A typical treatment course would require 12 to 18 months of residence within the therapeutic community, followed by day treatment support subsequent to gradua-tion. Few adolescents are able to tolerate prolonged con-finement in a therapeutic community and, even for those who stay, the prognosis following discharge is not good.

An alternative method of treatment for opiate addiction is methadone maintenance.[13] These treatment programs administer a daily dose of a substitute narcotic, metha-done, in combination with supportive services and be-havioral intervention. As methadone can be taken once daily by the oral route and has a more prolonged and less intense effect than heroin, clients in these programs can resume normal activities and pursue educational and vo-cational goals. The original hope that opiate addicts could thereby stabilize their lifestyles and eventually be detox-ified and remain abstinent has not been realized. Al-though many young people will achieve some success in remaining relatively drug-free while on methadone main-tenance, eventual detoxification and abstinence has been an overly optimistic goal. At the present time, methadone maintenance must be viewed as a potential lifelong ther-apy and hence should not be a treatment of first resort for most young people.

REFERENCES

1. Johnston LD, O'Malley PM, Bachman JG: *Drug Use by High School Seniors - The Class of 1986*, US Department of Health and Human Services publication No. (ADM) 87-1535. Rockville, MD, 1987
2. Simon EJ: Recent developments in the biology of opiates: Possible relevance to addiction, in Lowinson JH and Ruiz P (eds):*Substance Abuse: Clinical Problems and Perspectives*, Baltimore, Williams & Wilkins, 1981, pp 45-56

3. Easom JM, Lovejoy FH Jr: Opiates, in Haddad LM and Winchester JF (eds): *Clinical Management of Poisoning and Drug Overdose,* Philadelphia, WB Saunders, 1983, pp 424-433
4. Schonberg SK, Litt IF, Cohen MI: Drug Abuse, in Rudolph AM, Hoffman JIE (eds): *Pediatrics, 18th Edition,* Norwalk, Appleton & Lange, 1987, pp 745-758
5. United States Aids Program: *AIDS Weekly Surveillance Report,* Center for Infectious Disease, Centers for Disease Control, Atlanta, Georgia, February 29, 1988
6. Dreyer NP, Fields BN: Heroin associated infective endocarditis. *Ann Intern Med* 1973; 78:699-702
7. Cherubin CE: A review of the medical complications of narcotics addiction. *Int J Addict* 1968; 3:163-175
8. Litt IF, Cohen MI, Schonberg SK, et al: Liver disease in the drug-using adolescent. *J Pediatr* 1972; 81:238-242
9. Brown SM, Stimmel B, Taub RN, et al: Immunologic dysfunction in heroin addicts. *Arch Intern Med* 1974; 134:1001-1006
10. Stoffer SS: A gynecologic study of drug addicts. *Am J Obstet Gynecol* 1968; 101:779-783
11. Jaffe JJ, Martin WR: Opioid analgesics and antagonists, in Gilman AG, Goodman LS, Rall TW, et al (eds): *The Pharmacological Basis of Therapeutics,* New York, Macmillan, 1985, pp 491-531
12. Madden JD, Chappel JN, Zuspan F, et al: Observation and treatment of neonatal narcotic withdrawal. *Am J Obstet Gynecol* 1977; 127:199-201
13. Rosenberg CM, Patch VD: Methadone use in adolescent heroin addicts. *JAMA,* 1972; 220:991-993

SEDATIVES/HYPNOTICS

1. EPIDEMIOLOGY

Among the sedative/hypnotic drugs subject to abuse are the barbiturates, such as phenobarbital and secobarbital ("reds"), amobarbital ("blues") and pentobarbital ("yellow jackets"), as well as methaqualone ("ludes" or "soapers") and glutethimide ("goofballs"). Ethinamate and methyprylon are other drugs designed to promote sleep that have potential for toxicity, addiction, and abuse. Approximately 10% of high school seniors in 1986 reported some lifetime use of a sedative/hypnotic.[1]

Barbiturates were first used in medical practice at the beginning of the twentieth century. Although they are still widely prescribed, they have been largely supplanted by the benzodiazepines and other drugs in their role as sedatives. Methaqualone was introduced into the United States in 1965 and was touted to be a safe, nonaddicting, nonbarbiturate with a low potential for abuse. These claims were soon proved to be far from accurate. In fact, methaqualone clearly did cause physical dependence, and it rapidly became a major drug of abuse, having earned a reputation for producing a greater "high" than the barbiturates and for being an aphrodisiac. Although methaqualone is now a Schedule II drug and most manufacturers have suspended production, "bootleg" forms are still available.

2. PHARMACOLOGY

Barbituric acid, a substance with no central nervous system (CNS) activity itself, is the parent compound for all the barbiturates. The degree of lipid solubility varies among the barbiturates, with more rapid onset, shorter duration of action, and greater degree of hypnotic activity being associated with the more lipid-soluble compounds. Barbiturates are classified as long-acting, 12-24 hours (e.g., phenobarbital); intermediate-acting, 8-10 hours (e.g., amobarbital); short-acting, 4-8 hours (e.g., pentobarbital); and, ultra-short acting, 3-4 hours (e.g., thiopental).

All of the barbiturates are rapidly absorbed after oral ingestion or subcutaneous injection, after which they are either detoxified in the liver or excreted unchanged in the urine. Elimination is delayed in infants, pregnant women, and patients with diminished renal or hepatic function. The barbiturates exert their action on the CNS by depressing synaptic responses, delaying the synaptic recovery, and decreasing postsynaptic resistance. Because of their high lipid solubility, the rapidly acting barbiturates are quickly taken up by the gray matter, which is quite vascular, and sleep is induced within minutes. Methaqualone is rapidly and completely absorbed after oral ingestion, reaching peak levels within one to two hours. It is metabolized in the liver to inactive forms that are excreted in the urine. Glutethimide is slowly and erratically absorbed after oral use, except when it is taken with alcohol, which dramatically increases the rate of absorption. It is highly lipid soluble and becomes distributed into brain and adipose tissue rapidly. Most of the drug is detoxified by the liver, with less than 2% excreted unchanged in the urine.

3. HEALTH CONSEQUENCES

The CNS effects of the sedative/hypnotic drugs range from mild sedation to general anesthesia. All of these drugs produce some level of drowsiness, although tolerance to this effect develops over time. The individual who abuses barbiturates will often display slurred speech, a short attention span, emotional lability, nystagmus, and ataxia.[2] Methaqualone produces effects that may be mistaken for alcohol inebriation. Patients will have slurred speech, an unsteady gait, impaired judgment, and poor impulse control.[3] The user of glutethimide and other non-barbiturate sedatives/hypnotics may exhibit sedation as well as the effects described above.[2] While intoxicated, the abuser of sedatives/hypnotics is at risk of trauma as well as subject to poor performance at school or at work.

While tolerance to the physical and psychological effects does occur at normal doses, no tolerance develops to an acute lethal dose, thus making overdose common. In patients suffering from acute intoxication, the barbiturates exert their depressive effects on a variety of systems. One manifestation is obtundation, ranging from drowsiness to coma; this may be followed by respiratory and cardiovascular collapse and death. Pulmonary edema and aspiration pneumonia are occasionally encountered. Miosis, diminished or absent pupillary and corneal reflexes, abnormal temperature regulation (hypothermia occurring early, with hyperthermia occurring later), and decreased gastrointestinal motility with delayed gastric emptying time are also seen.[4]

Overdose with methaqualone may cause features that are quite different from those produced by the other sedatives/hypnotics including increased deep tendon reflexes, muscular hypertonicity, myoclonus, generalized muscle twitching, shivering, and occasionally, seizures.[5] Severe toxicity will produce coma, respiratory depression, and increased vascular permeability, resulting in effusions and pulmonary edema. The symptoms of glutethimide intoxication are similar to those of the barbiturates, except that there are often cyclic fluctuations in the depth of the coma, which can be prolonged. Because glutethimide acts as an anticholinergic, mydriasis, urinary retention, thick, tenacious secretions, and dry mouth may also occur.

Other somatic consequences are secondary to the intravenous abuse of sedatives. Tablets and capsules are dissolved in water and injected under unsterile conditions and frequently contaminated with particulate material. Infections such as cellulitis, subcutaneous abscesses, and hepatitis, as well as talc and starch granulomata and emboli in the lung, may develop in such cases. The latter may subsequently produce pulmonary hypertension.

The sedative/hypnotic drugs are highly addictive. The dose and period of use necessary to induce tolerance and addiction vary with each barbiturate. On the average, however, addiction develops within one to two months of regular daily use of 500 mg or more. Addiction to methaqualone has been reported in adults after the use of 2 grams daily for as little as one month.[5] Glutethimide and all of the other nonbarbiturate sedatives produce tolerance and addiction with persistent use.

The abstinence syndrome with the sedative/hypnotics is quite serious and in fact can be life-threatening. Anxiety, restlessness, tremors, insomnia, abdominal cramps, nausea, and vomiting are the earliest symptoms of withdrawal. These usually begin between 12-16 hours after the last dose of a short-acting barbiturate or glutethimide. By 24 hours, the patient has hyperactive reflexes and orthostatic hypotension. If left untreated, symptoms peak at 48-72 hours, with the onset of hallucinations, delirium, and generalized seizures.[6] The longer- acting barbiturates are associated with the same reaction pattern, but the symptoms are delayed. Seizures may not occur until one week after the last dose.

Withdrawal symptoms occur after three to five days of abstinence in the individual who is addicted to methaqualone. Symptoms include headache, anorexia, abdominal cramps, abnormal sleep patterns, and in the most severe cases, seizures.[5]

The barbiturates freely cross the placenta, resulting in equal maternal and fetal plasma concentrations. Because elimination is increased during pregnancy, however, lower plasma levels result. Fetal abnormalities have been reported with barbiturate use during pregnancy.[7] Withdrawal symptoms may occur in neonates born to women who use these drugs during the third trimester of pregnancy.[8,9] Little is known regarding consequences to the fetus of a woman who has used methaqualone or glutethimide during pregnancy.

4. LABORATORY EVALUATION

Plasma and urine testing is widely available for the qualitative and quantitative detection of barbiturates. Most medical facilities routinely use such testing to determine therapeutic levels of these drugs and are able to supply the information needed to diagnose suspected abuse or a drug overdose (See Chapter 4).

5. TREATMENT CONSIDERATIONS

The objective of the initial management of a patient who has taken a toxic overdose of a sedative/hypnotic drug is to prevent further absorption of the drug. This is of particular importance since gastrointestinal motility is reduced in these patients, allowing continued absorption for hours or even days. An alert patient who is being treated soon after an ingestion may be given ipecac syrup. This is followed by administration of activated charcoal and then a saline cathartic, such as magnesium citrate. The comatose patient or one with any respiratory embarrassment will require intubation with a cuffed endotracheal tube to prevent aspiration and maintain a patent airway. Monitoring of serum electrolytes, blood gases, urinary output, and plasma barbiturate levels will help guide fluid replacement and other aspects of supportive therapy. For all the barbiturates, increasing urinary output is beneficial; alkalinization of the urine is also helpful with the long-acting barbiturates. Hemodialysis may be effective with the barbiturates and glutethimide, but it is rarely necessary. With glutethimide or methaqualone intoxication, fluid therapy must be judicious, as pulmonary edema may accompany poisoning. Vasopressors may be needed to treat hypotension.

Anticipation and treatment of the abstinence syndrome are essential. Any individual who has used 500 mg or more of barbiturates daily for at least one month and all patients with a history of a seizure disorder who use any amount of sedatives regularly, should undergo detoxification on an inpatient unit. Phenobarbital is used in gradually tapered doses until the patient is drug-free.[10] When seizures occur from barbiturate withdrawal, they will usually be unresponsive to phenytoin and must be treated with barbiturates. Chlorpromazine is contraindicated because of its tendency to lower the seizure threshold. The individual addicted to methaqualone should also be detoxified with phenobarbital, but it can be accomplished over a briefer period of time, usually within three to five days.[11]

REFERENCES

1. Johnston LD, O'Malley PM, Bachman JG: *Drug Use by High School Seniors - The Class of 1986*, US Department of Health and Human Services publication No. (ADM) 87-1535. Rockville, MD, 1987

2. Harvey SC: Hypnotics and sedatives, in Gilman AG, Goodman LS, Rall TW, et al (eds): *The Pharmacological Basis of Therapeutics*, New York, Macmillan, 1985, pp 339-371

3. Kulberg A: Substance abuse: Clinical identification and management. *Ped Clin North Am* 1986; 33:325-361
4. Winchester JF: Barbiturates, in Haddad LM, and Winchester JF (eds): *Clinical Management of Poisoning and Drug Overdose*, Philadelphia, WB Saunders, 1983, pp 413-424
5. Litovitz T: Methaqualone, in Haddad LM, and Winchester JF (eds): *Clinical Management of Poisoning and Drug Overdose*, Philadelphia, WB Saunders, 1983, pp. 466-469
6. Anon.: Barbiturates. *Clin Toxicol Rev* 1981; 3:No.10
7. Smith DW: Teratogenicity of anticonvulsive medications. *Am J Dis Child* 1977; 131:1337-1339
8. Desmond MM, Schwanecke RP, Wilson GS, et al: Maternal barbiturate utilization and neonatal withdrawal symptomatology. *J Pediatr* 1972; 80:190-197
9. Reveri M, Pyati SP, Pildes RS: Neonatal withdrawal symptoms associated with glutethimide (Doriden) addiction in the mother during pregnancy. *Clin Pediatr* 1977; 16:424-425
10. Smith DE, Wesson DR: Phenobarbital technique for treatment of barbiturate dependence. *Arch Gen Psychiatry* 1971; 24:56-60
11. Schonberg SK, Litt IF, Cohen MI: Drug abuse, in Rudolph AM, and Hoffman JIE (eds): *Pediatrics*, Norwalk, Conn., Appleton & Lange, 1987; pp 745-760

TRANQUILIZERS

1. EPIDEMIOLOGY

Tranquilizers, including the benzodiazepines and meprobamate, are the most prescribed group of drugs in the United States. There has been a relatively low but consistent rate of experimentation with and use of these drugs within the adolescent population;[1] more important, however, is that these drugs, particularly diazepam (Valium®), are widely prescribed and readily available to young people.

2. PHARMACOLOGY

While the pharmacokinetics of the benzodiazepines vary considerably, their other pharmacologic and toxic properties are quite similar and are a result of their effects on the central nervous system (CNS). After oral ingestion, the benzodiazepines are all readily and rapidly absorbed from the stomach. Whether they are used orally, intramuscularly, or intravenously, all the benzodiazepines become bound to plasma proteins once they enter the systemic circulation. The extent to which the drugs bind varies somewhat depending on their degree of lipid solubility; however, they tend to be widely distributed into body tissues.

The benzodiazepines undergo biotransformation in the liver; however, it is interesting to note that the elimination half-life and body clearance of a particular compound often do not reflect the duration of action of the drug. Recent evidence would indicate that the benzodiazepines indirectly exert their effect on the CNS by potentiating the effects of gamma-aminobutyric acid (GABA).[2] The muscle-relaxant effect of these drugs may be explained by the fact that GABA inhibits presynaptic neurons in the spinal cord.

Meprobamate is readily absorbed from the gastrointestinal tract, reaching a peak concentration within one to two hours after ingestion. Most of the drug is oxidized in the liver and excreted in the urine. Like the barbiturates, with which it shares many pharmacologic and clinical properties, meprobamate will over time induce microsomal enzymes, thereby speeding the metabolic disposition of other drugs that are affected by this form of enzymatic degradation.

3. HEALTH CONSEQUENCES
The benzodiazepines are potent anticonvulsants and muscle relaxants. Drowsiness, ataxia, dizziness, and weakness are common side effects, even at therapeutic doses. In addition, impairment of both psychomotor performance and memory can occur with their use.[3]

The benzodiazepines are effective for the treatment of anxiety and insomnia and they are prescribed frequently, more often in adults than adolescents, for this purpose. Until recently, diazepam was the most widely used prescription drug in the United States. Euphoria is a concommitant of rapid absorption, and explains the potential for abuse by teenagers.

The salient feature of benzodiazepine overdose is sedation. Other effects are paresthesias, blurred vision, dysarthria, and nystagmus. There is little or no effect on blood pressure and respiratory status when these drugs are used orally. Acute intoxication is more likely to occur when the benzodiazepines are taken with alcohol or other depressants than when the drugs are taken alone.[2] This is not only because the effects are additive but also because alcohol increases the rate of absorption of the benzodiazepines. Paradoxical reactions consisting of agitation and frightening hallucinations, although uncommon, do occur.

The benzodiazepines with a long half-life, such as diazepam or flurazepam, tend to produce cumulative sedation; however, this is partly offset by the development of tolerance. Physiological dependence does occur, and an abstinence syndrome may begin as long as five to eight days after the last dose of the longer half-life forms and continue for several weeks.[4] For those benzodiazepines with a relatively short half-life (e.g., oxazepam, lorazepam, alprazolam, or triazolam) the withdrawal syndrome begins more rapidly. The mildest symptoms of withdrawal are insomnia, sensitivity to light and sound, and irritability; these may progress to tremulousness, diaphoresis, muscle twitching, tachycardia, systolic hypertension, confusion, and convulsions.[5]

When meprobamate was released in the 1950s, it was promoted as a muscle relaxant; however, it has been found to be relatively ineffective for this purpose and is now mainly used as a tranquilizer and hypnotic. Allergic reactions, aplastic anemia, thrombocytopenia, leukopenia, agranulocytosis, and erythroid hypoplasia have all been associated with the use of meprobamate.[6] Meprobamate toxicity is manifested by vomiting, paresthesia, hemodynamic instability, coma, and convulsions. Profound and persistent hypotension as well as cardiac dysrhythmias may occur after large ingestions. An abstinence syndrome following abrupt cessation of chronic use of high doses of meprobamate is similar to barbiturate withdrawal and may include seizures, coma, and death.[7] Benzodiazepines cross the placenta and accumulate in the fetus. There is some evidence that their use during the first trimester of pregnancy may result in increased risk of oral clefts.[2] There have been reports of cardiac, brain, palate, and limb abnormalities in babies born to mothers who have used meprobamate during pregnancy, but a direct cause-and-effect relationship has not been proved.[8]

4. LABORATORY EVALUATION
The benzodiazepines and meprobamate can be measured in blood and urine (See Chapter 4).

5. TREATMENT CONSIDERATIONS
Treatment of overdose in the conscious patient consists of the administration of ipecac syrup to empty the stomach, the use of activated charcoal, followed by a cathartic such as magnesium citrate. If the patient is comatose or otherwise severely compromised, intubation, ventilation, and circulatory support may be necessary.

The abstinence syndrome is treated by reinstituting the benzodiazepine and slowly tapering dosage over a four to six week period.[9] In instances of addiction to meprobamate, that is when it is known or suspected that the patient has been taking large doses of meprobamate chronically (e.g., 3 gms or more daily for at least two months), either meprobamate or a barbiturate should be used for detoxification, proceeding as one would for barbiturate withdrawal.[10]

REFERENCES

1. Johnston LD, O'Malley PM, Bachman JG: *Drug Use by High School Seniors - The Class of 1986*, US Department of Health and Human Services publication No. (ADM) 87-1535. Rockville, MD 1987
2. Litovitz T: Benzodiazepines, in Haddad LM, Winchester JF (eds): *Clinical Management of Poisoning and Drug Overdose*, Philadelphia, WB Saunders, 1983, pp 475-482
3. Anon.: Choice of benzodiazepines. *Med Lett Drugs Ther* 1988;30:25-28

4. Kulberg A: Substance abuse: Clinical identification and management. *Pediatr Clin North Amer* 1986; 33:325-361
5. Mellor CS, Jain VK: Diazepam withdrawal syndrome: Its prolonged and changing nature. *Can Med Assoc J* 1982; 127:1093-1096
6. Katz RL: Drug therapy: Sedatives and tranquilizers. *N Engl J Med* 1972; 286:757-760
7. Harvey SC: Hypnotics and sedatives, in Gilman AG, Goodman LS, Rall TW, et al (eds): *The Pharmacological Basis of Therapeutics*, New York, Macmillan, 1985, pp 339-371
8. Milkovich L, van der Berg BJ: Effects of prenatal meprobamate and chlordiazepoxide hydrochloride on human embryonic and fetal development. *N Engl J Med* 1974; 291:1268-1271
9. Higgitt AC, Lader MH, Fonagy P: Clinical management of benzodiazepine dependence. *Br Med J* 1985; 291:688-690
10. Smith DE, Wesson DR: Phenobarbital technique for treatment of barbiturate dependence. *Arch Gen Psychiatry* 1971; 24:56-60

DESIGNER DRUGS

According to the estimate of the Drug Enforcement Administration (DEA), the newest billion dollar industry in the United States is designer drugs.[1] These are synthetic chemical modifications of extant drugs of abuse that are designed and manufactured in makeshift laboratories and sold at great profit for recreational use. The advantages to sellers and users are that most modified drugs are technically not illegal until they can be identified, evaluated, and placed on Schedule I or II by the DEA.[2] In addition, many designer drugs are stronger and cheaper than the substance from which they are derived.

DESIGNER OPIATES

Modifications of the drugs meperidine (Demerol®) and fentanyl came to attention on the West Coast in the late 1970s, when several unexplained deaths were traced to overdose of alpha-methylfentanyl.[3] This compound is a synthetic analogue of fentanyl citrate and is an exceedingly powerful opiate. The more recent derivative found on the illicit market is 3-methylfentanyl, a drug that is

2000 times as potent as morphine. In 1986, it had been responsible for at least 12 deaths in San Francisco.[1]

Sloppy and uncontrolled manufacturing processes pose great dangers to consumers of designer drugs. 1-methyl-4-phenyl-4-propionoxy-piperidine (MPPP) is a designer modification of meperidine. If the chemical synthetic process is not strictly controlled, however, a significant amount of a contaminant, 1-methyl-4-phenyl-1,2,5,6-tetrahydropyridine (MPTP) is formed. MPTP is a neurotoxin that has a predilection for the substantia nigra of the brain and causes irreversible Parkinson's disease.[4] The first designer drug catastrophe was identified in 1982, when a group of young drug addicts in California suddenly developed severe Parkinsonism due to this contaminant.

DESIGNER EUPHORIANTS

Two new drugs that are chemically related to both hallucinogens and stimulants have recently appeared. Called "Ecstasy" and "Eve," both drugs are modifications of methamphetamine. Ecstasy (3,4-methylenedioxymethamphetamine, or MDMA) began to be used legally by psychiatrists to facilitate psychotherapy in the 1970s.[5] Since 1983, it has become a recreational drug popular on college campuses. In July 1985, MDMA became a controlled substance and was placed on Schedule I by the DEA; however, it is still readily available on the illicit market. In oral doses of 100 mg, it is reported to induce euphoria and enhanced self-awareness. It does not induce hallucinations or visual perceptual distortions. In 1985, MDMA's legal replacement appeared on the street in the form of 3,4-methylenedioxyethamphetamine (MDEA, or Eve). This drug is reported to have effects similar to but milder than Ecstasy. In October 1987, MDEA also became a controlled substance and was placed on Schedule I by the DEA.

In a recent survey, 39% of a randomly selected group of 369 Stanford University students reported having used Ecstasy at least once, and many students had taken it five times or more.[6] To date, there is no documentation of use of these drugs by high school students, but it can only be a matter of time before such reports begin to appear.

While Ecstasy and Eve are thought to be quite safe by recreational users and by psychotherapists, a recent paper from Dallas has documented five deaths in association with them. The patients ranged in age from 18-32 years and included four men and one woman.[7] In three of the deaths, the drug may have contributed to the induction of arrhythmias in individuals with underlying cardiac or pulmonary disease. One death was apparently due to bizarre and risky behavior resulting in an accident. In the fifth person, MDMA was thought to be the immediate cause of death.

Many drug-abuse experts fear that the current situation with respect to designer drugs may only be the beginning of a much more serious problem. Once illicit marketeers begin chemical production in garages and kitchens across the country, the demand for imported botanically derived drugs may decrease and regulation of the flow of illicit drugs will be much more difficult.

REFERENCES

1.   Ziporyn T: A growing industry and menace: makeshift laboratory's designer drugs. *JAMA* 1986; 256(22):3061-3063

2.   Hagerty C: Designer Drug Enforcement Act seeks to attack problem at source. *Am Pharm* 1985; NS25(10):10-11

3.   Brittain JL: China white: the bogus drug. *J Toxicol Clin Toxicol* 1982; 19:1123-1126

4.   Langston JW: Parkinson's disease: current view. *Am Fam Physician* 1987; 35(3):201-206

5.   Clinko RP, Roehtich H, Sweeney DR, et al: Ecstasy: a review of MDMA and MDA. *Int J Psychiatry Med* 1986-87; 16(4):359-372

6.   Peroutka SJ: Incidence of recreational use of 3,4-methylenedioxymethamphetamine (MDMA, "Ecstasy") on an under-graduate campus. *N Engl Med* 1987; 317(24):1542-1543

7.   Dowling GP, McDonough III ET, Bost RO: 'Eve' and 'Ecstasy' a report of five deaths associated with the use of MDEA and MDMA. *JAMA* 1987; 257:1615-1617

Index

rights of adolescents in seeking
treatment for, 107-114
role of PCP in documenting suspected use, 42-47
symptoms of, 1
Drug use programs, alternatives to,
80
DUI (driving under influence) programs, 17, 96-98, 124

E

"Ecstasy," 181, 182
Edema, 165
Educator, role of primary care physi-
cian as, 26
"Elephant (Monkey) Tranquilizer,"
157
Emancipated minor, rights of con-
cerning health care, 105-106
Emphysema, and smoking, 118
Endocarditis, 164
infective, 165
Enzyme-multiple immunoassay tech-
nique (EMIT), 160
Enzyme-multiplied immunoassay
technique, 58
Eosinophilia, 41
Epinephrine, 145
Erythloxylon coca, 138
Ethical and legal considerations,
100-114
adolescents and health care, 104-
107
and confidentiality, 107-114
Ethinamate, 170
Ethnic minorities, gateway drug use
by, 3
Ethyl alcohol, 122
Evaluation, by interview, 34-47
"Eve," 181, 182

F

Families Anonymous (FA), 30, 76
Family
alcohol use in, 122
drug prevention programs focused on, 87-89
drug use as problem for, 24

responsibility of primary care
physicians to, 22-25
Family court, referral of cases con-
cerning medical neglect, 104
Family Court Act (Il., 1899), 100-
101
Family support groups, 76
Fenfluramine hydrochloride, 148
Fentanyl, modifications of, 180-181
Flashbacks
and LSD use, 155
and marijuana use, 133
Fluorescence polarization immunoas-
say, 58-59
Flurazepam, 178
Freebase, 137, 140
Freons, 145

G

Gamma-aminobutyric acid (GABA),
177
Gas chromatography, 60-61
Gas chromatography/mass spec-
trometry, 61
Gas-liquid chromatography, 160
Gasoline sniffing, 144, 145
Gastric lavage, 156
Gastrointestinal effects, of opiate
abuse, 165-166
Gateway drugs, 3
In re Gault, 102
Genetic factors, role of, in alco-
holism, 4-5
Glenn, H. Stephen, 88
Glue-sniffing, 145-146 *See also* In-
halants
Glutethimide, 170, 172
Glutethimide intoxication, 173
Government, involvement of local, in
drug abuse programs, 28

H

Hallucinations
from amphetamines, 150
from hallucinogens, 153-154
from inhalants, 145
Hallucinogens
adolescent use of, 152